Interpreting Obstetric Ultrasound

AF520230

Interpreting Obstetric Ultrasound

A CASE-BASED APPROACH

Amar Bhide
MD MRCOG
Consultant in Fetal Medicine
St. George's Hospital, London, UK

Universities Press

Universities Press (India) Private Limited

Registered Office
3-6-747/1/A & 3-6-754/1, Himayatnagar
Hyderabad 500 029 (A.P.), India
E-mail: info@universitiespress.com

Distributed by
Orient Blackswan Private Limited

Registered Office
3-6-752, Himayatnagar
Hyderabad 500 029 (A.P.), India

Other Offices
Bangalore / Bhopal / Bhubaneshwar / Chennai / Ernakulam / Guwahati
Hyderabad / Jaipur / Kolkata / Lucknow / Mumbai / New Delhi / Patna

© Universities Press (India) Private Limited 2009
First Published 2009

Cover and book design
© Universities Press (India) Private Limited 2009

ISBN: 978 81 7371 645 4

Typeset by
MacroTex Solutions
Chennai 600 088

Printed at
Orion Printers Private Limited
Hyderabad 500 004

Published by
Universities Press (India) Private Limited
3-6-747/1/A & 3-6-754/1, Himayatnagar
Hyderabad 500 029 (A.P.), India

This book has been published in good faith that the material provided by the author is original. Every effort has been made to ensure accuracy of material, but the publisher, printer and author are not responsible for any inadvertent error(s).

PREFACE

Clinical medicine is always interesting. No two cases are the same, and new research is changing existing practice all the time. Even so, there are certain themes that we all come across on a regular basis. This book is about these themes.

The particulars of a case may change, but the basic principles used to address each clinical situation remain fairly constant. It is not possible to address a given clinical problem without thoroughly understanding the underlying theory. I have made an attempt to unravel these principles with the use of case scenarios that are encountered in our daily practice.

This book is not a textbook of fetal medicine, and it does not claim to cover the subject. It is not about rare or uncommon problems either. There are many excellent reference texts available for that purpose. This book should be used to understand common clinical problems and the approaches to solving them. I have assumed a basic knowledge of Obstetrics and that of either performing or interpreting ultrasonography in pregnancy. Although ultrasound scanning in pregnancy is considered as a screening test for problems by the medical profession, it is largely looked upon as a means of reassurance by the parents. It should flag up concerns when appropriate, but should reassure in the large majority.

Most texts on ultrasonography in pregnancy are arranged by organ system. This is a good way to learn the subject from the beginning, without leaving any knowledge gaps. However, when we see a case, many systems may be involved. This book is based on clinical problems. In that sense, this follows the principles of 'problem-based learning'. As our knowledge and understanding advances, some parts of the text may become obsolete. The principles of management, however, rarely change once we have developed an understanding of the problem.

The practice of ultrasound scanning in pregnancy may vary depending on local tradition, expectations of parents and local laws. This book is largely based on my experiences in the health services in the United Kingdom. The information presented may have to be modified according to regional differences in other parts of the world. This book should be useful to practising obstetricians, ultrasonographers, radiologists and specialists in Maternal-Fetal Medicine. This should also help candidates preparing for the MRCOG examination, for the RCR/ RCOG diploma in Obstetric Ultrasound and for the special skills module in Fetal Medicine conducted by the Royal College of Obstetricians and Gynaecologists.

I am grateful to Universities Press, my publishers, who have made it possible for the book to reach you in print. I am grateful to my family for putting up with the time demands. The secret of the success of tertiary referral units in the United Kingdom is the high quality of scans performed in the referring units by sonographers. Over the years, I have received some excellent referrals. Indeed, the sonographers who perform routine scans are worth their weight in gold. My workplace, St. George's Hospital Fetal Medicine Unit, is progressive, forward-looking, and strives for excellence. I have enjoyed working here, and have always felt privileged and wanted.

Lastly, I am extremely grateful to all my patients who placed so much confidence in me and treated me as a human being and not as God. Their questions and expectations have kept me on my toes, and their appreciation has kept me going.

I would appreciate feedback regarding the book, and suggestions about how it could be improved, so I can incorporate these in future editions.

Amar Bhide
abhide@sgul.ac.uk

CONTENTS

DEDICATION

This book is dedicated to the prospective parents of unborn children, who consistently showed confidence in me, questioned me from time to time, provided me with feedback and helped me become a better clinician.

CHAPTER 1

INCREASED NUCHAL TRANSLUCENCY

Case: A 17-year-old girl underwent a routine ultrasound scan at 12 weeks. The crown–rump length corresponded to the length of gestation. However, the operator noted an increase in nuchal translucency (NT). Although the mother was young, the possibility of Down syndrome was raised.

Fetuses with Trisomy 21 (Down syndrome) are associated with increased tissue/fluid in the cervical region. This was first noticed in the second trimester of pregnancy and later in the first. In the second trimester, the space between the skull and the skin is termed nuchal thickness. In the first trimester, this space is echo-poor and is termed nuchal translucency. Measurement of NT is an accepted screening technique for the prenatal diagnosis of Down syndrome in several developed countries. The risk of Down syndrome increases with maternal age. However, many babies with Down syndrome are born to young mothers as well.

Technique

The technique of NT measurement has been well-documented. Transabdominal scanning is adequate in 95% of cases (Fig. 1.1). In others, a transvaginal scan may be necessary. All sonographers should be certified by the Fetal Medicine Foundation. To ensure that uniform results are obtained, the same criteria should be used:

- The crown–rump length (CRL) should be 45–84 mm (gestational age of 11 + 4 weeks to 13 + 6 weeks).

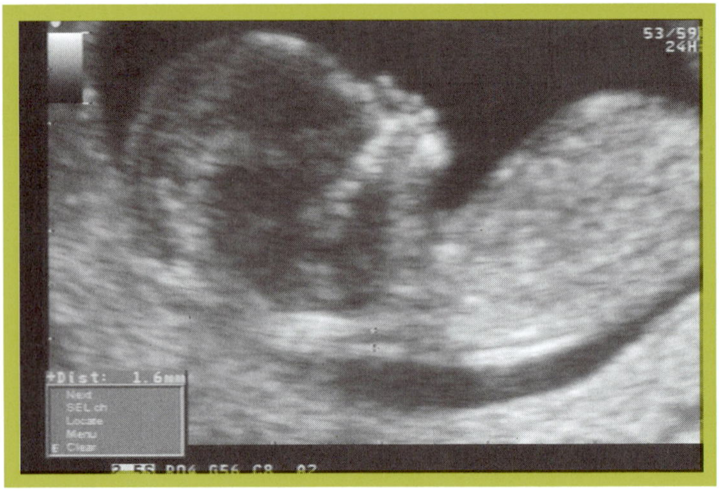

Figure 1.1: A fetus with normal NT

- A good sagittal section of the fetus should be obtained.
- The magnification should be such that the fetus occupies at least three-fourths of the screen.
- Care should be taken to distinguish the skin from the amnion. This is achieved by fetal movement away from the amniotic membrane.
- The maximum thickness of the space should be measured, multiple measurements taken, and the largest considered valid.
- Measurements should be taken in the neck 'neutral' position.
- If the umbilical cord is wound around the fetal neck, and measurements differ above and below the cord, the smaller measurement should be considered.

The Fetal Medicine Foundation audits the performance and takes into account the image quality as well as distribution of NT measurements. The image quality is assessed on appropriate magnification, section (sagittal or oblique), caliper placement, skin line and visualisation of the amnion separate from the nuchal membrane.

NT and Chromosomal Abnormalities

There have been reports of the association of fetal trisomy with increased NT at 11–14 weeks (Fig. 1.2).

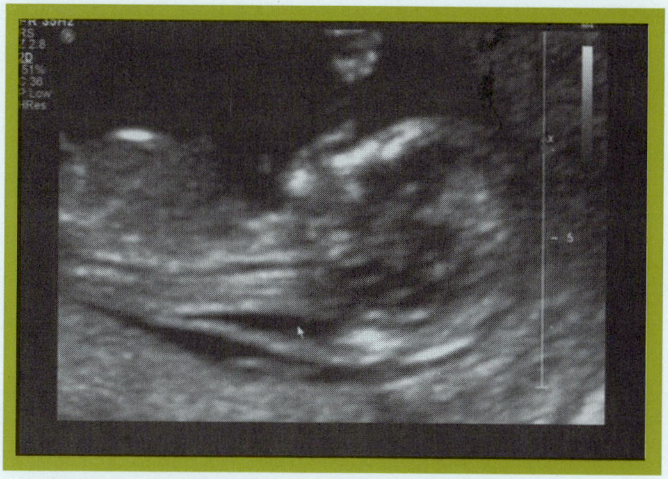

Figure 1.2: A fetus with increased NT

Initial reports used a fixed NT measurement of above 3 mm as the definition of abnormal. However, it was soon realised that NT measurement increases with gestational age. So an NT measurement over the 95th or 99th centile is increasingly being used to define abnormality (Fig. 1.3).

In the majority of cases, chromosomal abnormality involves chromosomes 21, 18, 13 or X (88% in a UK multicentre study). The higher the NT, the greater the risk of aneuploidy. The risk of a chromosomal abnormality is also linked to maternal age. The combination of maternal age and NT, with or without serum biochemistry, has been used to adjust the risk of aneuploidy for an individual pregnancy. The adjustments involve complex mathematical calculations and are best performed using a computer programme made available by the Fetal Medicine Foundation. NT measurements have been successfully used in a population screening programme for Down syndrome, and with maternal age, have been shown to detect 80% of cases of Down syndrome at a 5% screen-positive rate. The addition of serum biochemistry makes the test more effective. The current guidelines in the UK are to use a test that is at least 80% sensitive at a 3% screen-positive rate.

It has now been accepted that the nasal bone is not seen on ultrasound scans in 50–60% of fetuses with Down syndrome in the first trimester. The debate appears to be about what proportion of normal fetuses also fail to exhibit a nasal bone. The nasal bone remains hypoplastic in a significant proportion of fetuses with Down syndrome

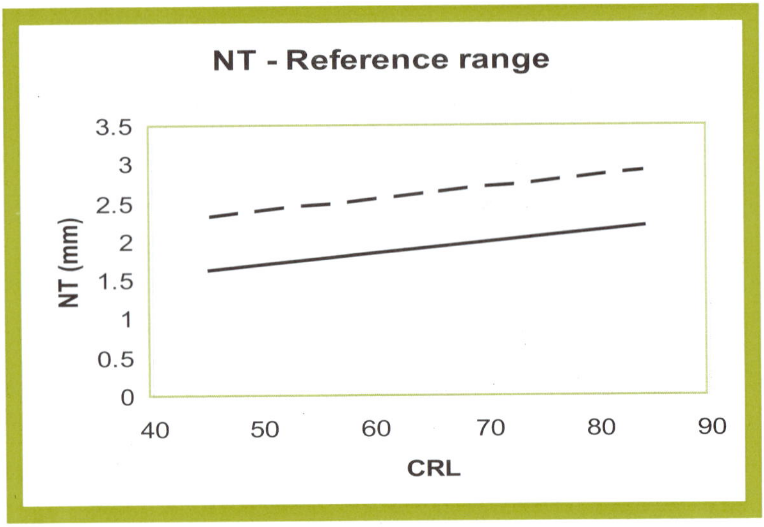

Figure 1.3: Mean (continuous line) and the 95th centile (dashed line) of NT for gestational age in Asian fetuses

even in the second trimester. This information can be used to further refine the risk of a fetus for Down syndrome. If the nasal bone is not visualised, the risk of Down syndrome would be higher. On the other hand, the risk would be reduced if the nasal bone is seen on the ultrasound scan. Absence of the nasal bone alone cannot be used to predict the risk; it should be determined in conjunction with NT.

Blood flow pattern in the ductus venosus has also been correlated with Down syndrome. Obtaining a Doppler signal from the ductus venosus in the first trimester is not too difficult. Absent or reversed 'a' wave or an increase in ductus venosus pulsatility (PIV) greater than the 95th centile is associated with increased risk of Down syndrome. Figure 1.4 shows a normal flow pattern through the ductus venosus while Fig. 1.5 shows a reversed 'a' wave.

Presence of tricuspid regurgitation in the fetal heart has also been correlated with Down syndrome. The Fetal Medicine Foundation has standardised the technique used to check for tricuspid regurgitation. It is recommended that pulsed wave technology be used, and that the regurgitation jet have a peak flow velocity of at least 60 cm/sec for it to be significant.

Following identification of increased NT, detection of a chromosomal abnormality requires a definitive test. The test of choice is often chorionic villus sampling, but this technique carries a miscarriage risk of approximately 1%. In a large series, the observed odds of being affected given a positive result (OAPR) were 1:10.

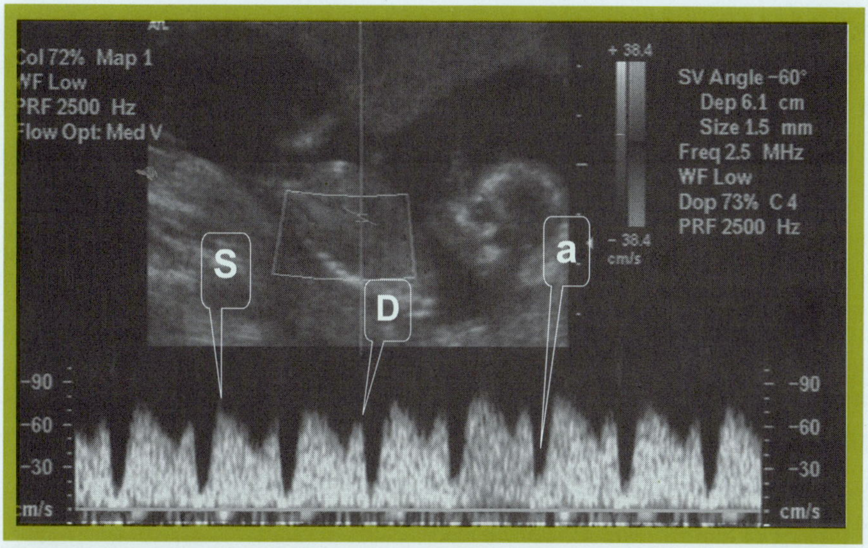

Figure 1.4: Normal flow velocity waveform through the ductus venosus. The components of the waveform have been labelled.

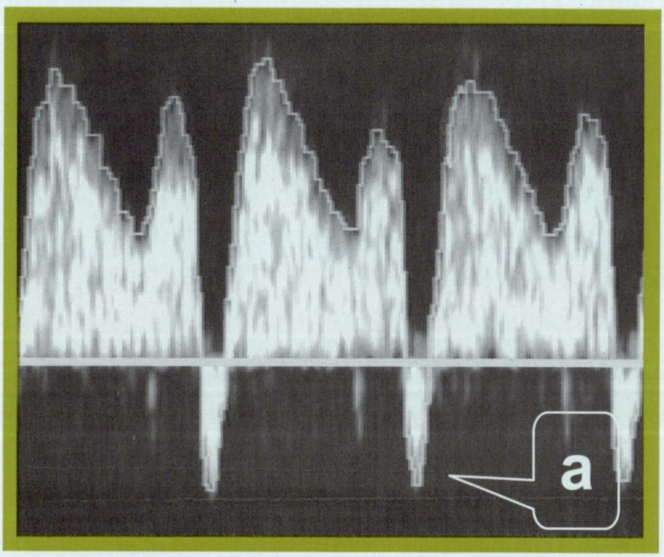

Figure 1.5: Reversed 'a' wave in the ductus venosus flow velocity waveform. The risk of a chromosomal abnormality is increased.

Increased NT and Normal Karyotype

Increased NT at 11–14 weeks is associated with a wide range of fetal abnormalities apart from chromosomal defects. The rates of miscarriage and perinatal death also rise in fetuses with increased NT. Michaelides and Economides reported that among fetuses with an NT greater than the 99th centile, 17.8% experienced adverse pregnancy outcome (termination for fetal abnormality, miscarriage or intrauterine death) as compared to 1.5% in those with a normal NT measurement. The congenital abnormality was detected only after birth in 6% of fetuses with increased NT (Table 1.1).

Several groups of **congenital abnormalities** have been linked with increase in NT. They can be grouped as follows:

- *Congenital heart defects (CHD):* NT is known to be associated with increased risk of congenital heart defects. The likelihood ratio for congenital heart disease with NT≥2.5 mm and ≥3.5 mm was 4.4 and 14.1, respectively. In general, this was found to be a poor screening test, with only 15% of major congenital heart defects associated with increased NT. The implication of this finding is that prevalence of CHD in fetuses with NT≥3.5 mm is 1:20 and detailed fetal echocardiography is indicated.
- *Fetal skeletal dysplasias*: Lethal skeletal dysplasias are associated with increased NT, probably as a result of fetal thoracic compression.
- *Fetal akinesia syndrome*: This is a heterogeneous group of conditions characterised by multiple joint contractures and abnormal motility. This group is frequently associated with fetal myopathy, neuropathy or underlying connective tissue abnormality.
- *Hematological abnormalities/Lymphatic defects:* Examples of these are alpha thalassemia and Fanconi's anemia. NT is increased in these conditions, possibly because of fetal anemia.

Table 1.1: Outcome of fetuses with increased NT and normal karyotype

NT	Adverse Pregnancy Outcome
<4.5 mm	10%
4.5–6.5 mm	20%
>6.5 mm	55%

- *Diaphragmatic hernia*: Compression of the intrathoracic structures from the herniated viscera is the likely explanation for increased NT.

The possible **mechanisms** include:

- Cardiac failure in association with abnormalities of the heart and great arteries
- Venous congestion in the head and neck in association with constriction of the fetal body in amnion rupture sequence, superior mediastinal compression found in diaphragmatic hernia, or narrow chest in skeletal dysplasia
- Failure of lymphatic drainage due to impaired fetal movement in various neuromuscular disorders
- Abnormal or delayed development of the lymphatic system
- Altered composition of subcutaneous connective tissue

Further Reading

- Jou HJ, SC Wu, TC Li, HC Hsu, CY Tzeng and FJ Hsieh. 2001. Relationship between fetal nuchal translucency and crown–rump length in an Asian population. *Ultrasound Obstet Gynecol* 17:111–14.
- Maverides E, F Cobian-Sanchez, A Tekay, G Moscoso, S Campbell, B Thilaganathan and JS Carvalho. 2001. Limitations of using first-trimester nuchal translucency measurement in routine screening for major congenital heart defects. *Ultrasound Obstet Gynecol* 17:106–10.
- Michaelides G and D Economides. 2001. Nuchal translucency measurement and pregnancy outcome in karyotypically normal fetuses. *Ultrasound Obstet Gynecol* 17:102–105.
- Nicolaides K, NJ Sebire and RJM Snijders (eds). 1999. The 11–14 week scan. The diagnosis of fetal abnormalities. Diploma in Fetal Medicine series. Parthenon Publishing.

Further Reading

- Snijders RJ, P Noble, N Sebire, A Souka and KH Nicolaides. 1998. UK multicentre project on assessment of risk of trisomy 21 by maternal age and fetal nuchal translucency thickness at 10–14 weeks of gestation. *Lancet* 351:343–46.

CHAPTER 2

TWIN GESTATION AND INVASIVE TESTING

Case: A 37-year-old woman underwent routine ultrasound scan at 12 weeks. The presence of a twin pregnancy was noticed. The parents requested prenatal diagnosis, as their previous baby had been diagnosed with beta thalassemia, and both the parents were carriers.

Multiple pregnancies constitute 1–2% of all pregnancies, with approximately 98% of such pregnancies comprising twin gestations. The use of assisted reproductive techniques and higher maternal age at conception are responsible for the increased prevalence of multiple pregnancies. As a consequence, these parents are likely to be less inclined to opt for any invasive testing because of the fear of pregnancy loss.

Many complicating features make twin pregnancies unique as far as prenatal diagnosis is concerned. It has now been established that it is the chorionicity and not the zygocity that determines the risk of specific complications. Chorionicity, accurate identification (numbering) of the twins and the prospect of discrepancies in the diagnosis of abnormality with possible selective reduction are three important factors to be considered.

Embryology of Monochorionic Twins

Monochorionic twins are derived from a single embryo, which subsequently divides. If division occurs early (within four days of fertilisation), each twin has its own chorion (dichorionic twins). These twins are indistinguishable from dizygotic dichorionic twins on ultrasound scan. If the division occurs on Day 9, not only the placenta but also the amniotic sac is shared (monoamniotic twins). Division after 10 days will lead to conjoined twins.

Chorionicity and Zygocity

Two-thirds of twin pregnancies are dizygotic, with one-third being monozygotic. Monochorionic pregnancies are necessarily monozygotic but dichorionic pregnancies may be mono or dizygotic. Accurate determination of chorionicity can be made using ultrasound scan, but this is reliable only in the first trimester. Figures 2.1 and 2.2 show the ultrasound method of determining chorionicity.

The presence of a 'lambda' or 'twin peak' sign is a reliable indicator of dichorionicity. Absence of this sign is indicative of monochorionicity in early pregnancy. After the first trimester, determination of chorionicity based on the lambda sign becomes increasingly unreliable. Presence of discordant genders and two clearly separate placental masses are indicators of dichorionicity. In a monochorionic twin pregnancy, individual sampling of the twins is unnecessary, as both will have the same genetic material.

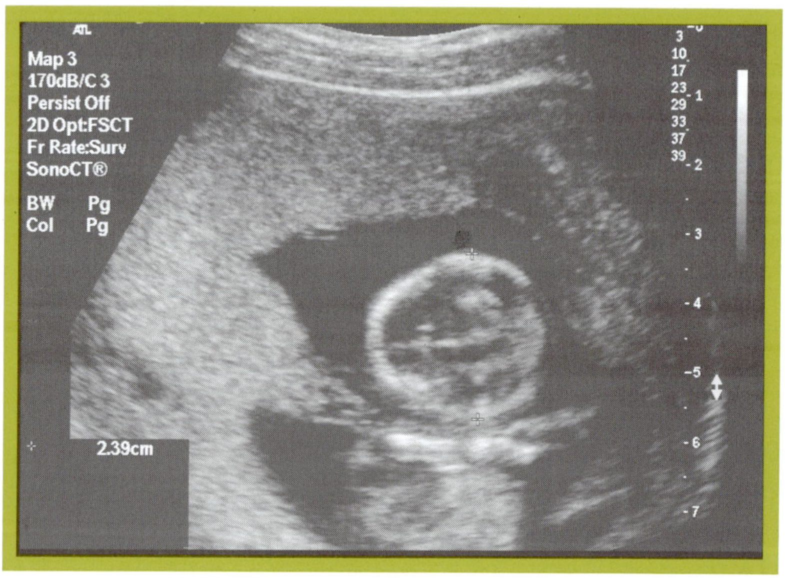

Figure 2.1: The 'lambda' or 'twin peak' sign, which is a reliable indicator of dichorionicity

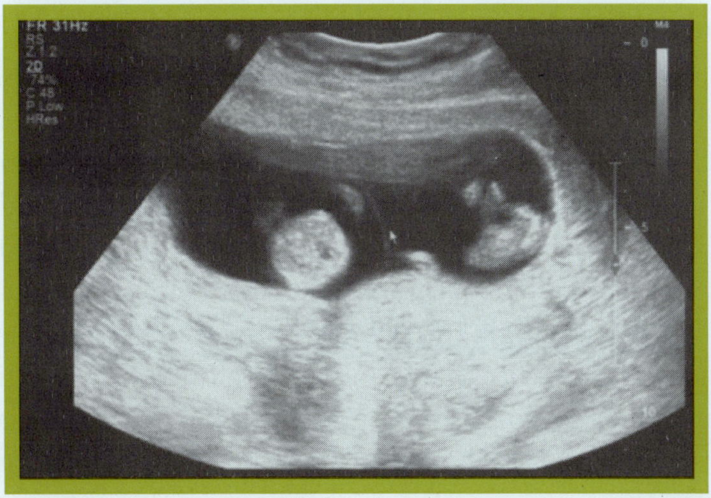

Figure 2.2: Absence of the 'lambda' or 'twin peak' sign (see arrow); note the thin membrane.

Numbering of Fetuses

The numbering of fetuses in a twin pregnancy is very important for easy identification of the individual fetus for serial examinations during the pregnancy. The convention followed is to use the relationship of the amniotic sac to the internal os. The fetus in the amniotic sac closest to the internal os is numbered fetus 1 and the ones farther away are numbered serially. Clear documentation of numbering is made on the first ultrasound scan. Once a number has been assigned early in the pregnancy, the same sequence is followed throughout the pregnancy.

Prospect of Discrepancies in the Diagnosis of Abnormality

Fetal karyotyping requires invasive testing by amniocentesis or chorionic villus sampling. Selection of the appropriate invasive technique depends on the reliability of the test and the procedure-related risk of fetal loss. Additionally, prenatal diagnosis of inheritable disease as well as chromosomal abnormality in multiple pregnancy is complicated by the possibility of obtaining discordant results. This possibility should be raised in the discussion leading to the decision to perform invasive testing. Selective termination or loss of a healthy co-fetus in the case of pregnancy loss might be unacceptable to some parents and the decision to undergo invasive testing may need to be modified.

Chorionic Villus Sampling

For a singleton pregnancy, chorionic villus sampling (CVS) may be performed transabdominally, transvaginally or with a combined abdominal–vaginal technique. CVS is not safe before 10 weeks (10 + 0). The transabdominal double-needle technique is a popular method. Great care should be taken in appropriate documentation of the samples to avoid incorrect identification of the individual twin. Furthermore, CVS in twins is complicated by the possibility of either sampling the same twin twice or contamination of cells from one placental mass with that of the other in fused dichorionic placentae, seen in about 5% of persons. To ensure that both fetuses are sampled, two entries are used—one for each placenta or for each of the extreme ends of a fused placenta. This precaution helps avoid contamination from the co-twin. de Catte et al reported the largest series so far, comprising 262 women with twin pregnancy having CVS; the loss rate was 5.5%. Out of 524 fetuses, 519 (99.05%) were sampled adequately.

Amniocentesis

Amniocentesis is not safe before 14 weeks (14 + 0). Both the sacs require sampling in twin amniocentesis. Amniocentesis can be carried out using the double-needle (one needle for each sac) or single-needle technique. 1 ml of amniotic fluid for every week of gestation (up to a maximum of 20 ml) is collected from each sac. Originally, a dye was placed in one of the amniotic sacs to avoid accidental sampling of the same sac twice. However, with reports of fetal intestinal atresia being linked with the use of methylene blue and the advent of real-time ultrasound scans, dyes are now rarely used. There has been no documented fetal risk with the use of indigo carmine.

Sebire et al described a technique for single-needle amniocentesis in multiple pregnancy. A careful ultrasound examination is first performed to note the viability, size, gender and position of each fetus, the placental site and the umbilical cord, and the location of the placental insertion of the inter-twin membrane. In the single-operator technique, the ultrasound probe held in the left hand of the operator is used to identify the site of insertion of the needle, ideally free of placental insertion and perpendicular to the amniotic membrane. After cleaning the appropriate site for with an antiseptic solution, a 20/21-gauge needle with a stylet is introduced into one of the amniotic sacs. The first 1 ml of the sample is discarded to avoid possible maternal contamination and the desired volume (usually 1 ml/week of gestation) of amniotic fluid is aspirated in a separate syringe. The stylet is replaced and the needle is then advanced through the inter-twin membrane into the other amniotic sac. The stylet is withdrawn and the desired volume is again aspirated after discarding the initial 1 ml to avoid contamination from the first twin. It is extremely important to label the samples accurately. In higher-order multiple pregnancies, the site of each amniotic sac and placental insertion must be carefully mapped and noted.

Yukobowich et al reported on 476 women with dichorionic twin pregnancy requiring amniocentesis and compared them with twin controls and singleton amniocentesis. The fetal loss rate after twin amniocentesis was higher (2.73%) than that for twin controls (0.63%) and singleton amniocentesis (0.6%).

Management options in multiple pregnancies where one of the fetuses is abnormal include expectant management, termination of the entire pregnancy or selective termination of the affected fetus. To a greater extent, the risk to the healthy fetus/fetuses should be evaluated before considering the outlook for the affected fetus. In case of uncertain chorionicity, invasive prenatal diagnosis should involve sampling of both fetuses. However, in terms of management for discordant fetal malformation, these pregnancies must be considered monochorionic and hence selective feticide using lethal injection is contraindicated because of the shared placental circulation.

Further Reading

- Bhide A and B Thilaganathan. 2004. Prenatal diagnosis in multiple pregnancy. *Best Pract Res Clin Obstet Gynaecol* 18:531–42.
- de Catte L, I Liebaers and W Foulon. 2000. Outcome of twin gestations after first trimester chorionic villus sampling. *Obstet Gynecol* 96:714–20.

Further Reading

- Sebire NJ, PL Noble, A Odibo et al. 1996. Single uterine entry for genetic amniocentesis in twin pregnancies. *Ultrasound Obstet Gynecol* 7:26–31.
- Yukobowich E, EY Anteby, SM Cohen et al. 2001. Risk of fetal loss in twin pregnancies undergoing second trimester amniocentesis. *Obstet Gynecol* 98:231–34.

CHAPTER 3
ANHYDRAMNIOS

Case: A 24-year-old woman in her first pregnancy underwent a routine anomaly scan at 22 weeks. The visualisation was difficult, but there was complete anyhdramnios. Fetal heart activity was detected, and the mother reported perceiving normal fetal movement.

Amniotic fluid dynamics has not been completely understood, but there are some well-known basic principles. After 16–18 weeks, amniotic fluid is produced mainly by fetal urination, with contributions from the lungs and across the walls of the blood vessels in the placenta. Amniotic fluid is removed by fetal swallowing; some of it is lost across the fetal membranes in the circulation as well. Fetal swallowing does not appear to be a significant factor before 26–28 weeks.

Technique of Measuring Amniotic Fluid Volume

In this standardised technique, it is recommended that the pregnant uterus be arbitrarily divided into four quadrants by an imaginary vertical line passing through the umbilicus, and another imaginary horizontal line passing mid-way between the symphysis pubis and the top of the uterine fundus. The maximum vertical height of the amniotic fluid pocket should be measured, making sure that the transducer is perpendicular to the skin. Loops of the umbilical cord are best excluded. The sum of the amniotic fluid measured in the four quadrants is designated as the amniotic fluid index (AFI). Inability to identify any pool of liquor without the umbilical cord is called anhydramnios.

Anhydramnios at this stage of pregnancy is associated with a guarded outcome regardless of the underlying etiology. The three causes are preterm prelabour rupture of membranes (PPROM), renal abnormality and severe early onset fetal growth restriction

Preterm Prelabour Rupture of Membranes (PPROM)

A good history is invaluable. Often, there is a history of loss of fluid in a gush, which has since reduced. This history is suggestive of membrane rupture. Although all the fluid may have drained off, it is produced on a continuous basis, and vaginal loss will not cease completely. The loss of liquor may not be appreciated if simultaneous vaginal bleeding is also seen.

The main problems are spontaneous preterm labour and development of chorioamnionitis. Once the membranes are ruptured, there is a significant risk that labour may start. Approximately half the women who undergo PPROM at this stage of pregnancy will remain undelivered two weeks later. After the first two weeks, the risk of preterm labour is relatively less. No effective interventions to reduce the risk of labour are available.

Development of chorioamnionitis is dependant on the gestational age at membrane rupture and the duration. Severe preterm PROM is likely to be infection driven. The longer the mother is undelivered, the higher the risk of infection. However, if infection has not set in in the initial two weeks, the chance that it will set in later is reduced. There is no evidence of any beneficial effect from the use of prophylactic antibiotics.

The diagnosis of chorioamnionitis is often clinical. The signs include presence of maternal pyrexia, general feeling of being unwell, uterine tenderness and presence of offensive liquor. Of these, the commonest and least subjective is maternal pyrexia. Increasing white cell count and higher levels of maternal C-reactive protein are supportive signs, but they are not specific enough for definitive ruling in or out of infection. White cell count may be elevated as a response to maternal steroid administration.

Normal amniotic fluid volume between 16 and 24 weeks' pregnancy is essential for normal lung development. Lack of amniotic fluid in this crucial interval may lead to pulmonary hypoplasia (Fig. 3.1). The risk is approximately 40%. In most cases, lung hypoplasia is an all-or-nothing phenomenon; so survival with compromised lung function is uncommon. Preterm PROM may be followed by prompt delivery of a pre-viable fetus with subsequent fetal demise.

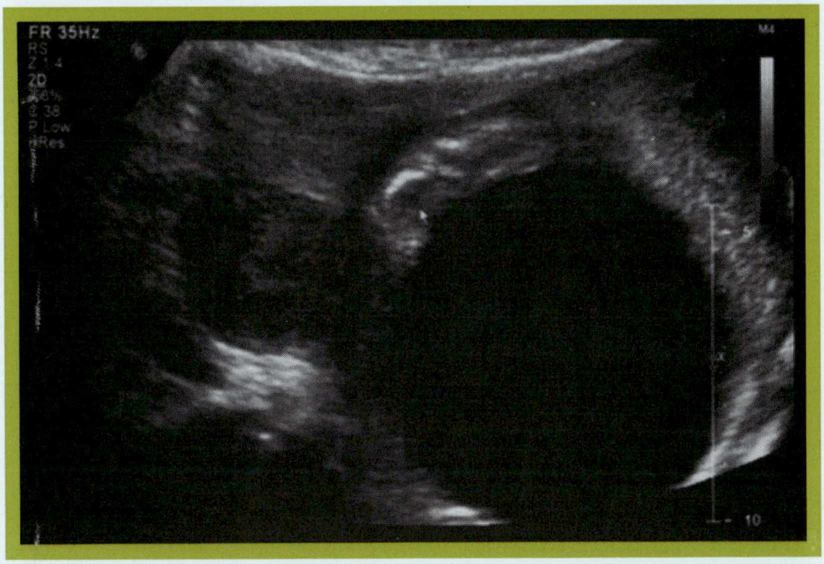

Figure 3.1: Megacystis in this fetus; note the absence of amniotic fluid around this fetus.

If the pregnancy can be prolonged to reasonable maturity but the lungs do not develop, the same end result is expected. On the other hand, if the lungs are developed, the baby will do well. A third alternative is severe prematurity and normal lung development. Survival of the baby but with severe handicap due to prematurity is possible. This should be explained to the parents while choosing a conservative option for the management of such pregnancies. Delivery should take place at a unit capable of looking after preterm babies who may require ventilatory support.

Renal Abnormality

The most common renal abnormality responsible for anhydramnios is bilateral renal agenesis. Diagnosis is based on the finding of anhydramnios and persistent failure to visualise the urinary bladder. The lack of amniotic fluid impairs image quality significantly. Visualisation of the kidneys should not be relied upon, as enlarged adrenal glands can be mistaken for the kidneys. Colour flow mapping to view the renal arteries has been suggested. However, it is of academic interest, since even if the presence of kidneys can be demonstrated, urine production does not take place. The outlook for the fetus is very guarded. Again, lethal lung hypoplasia is inevitable and is the cause of death after birth

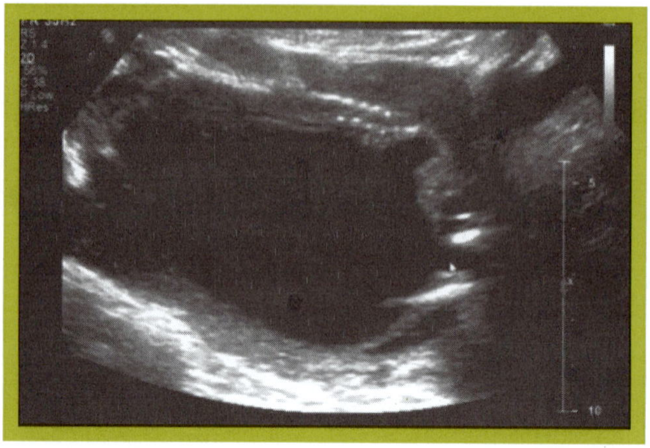

Figure 3.2: Fetal obstructive uropathy; the arrow shows the dilated posterior urethra. The fetal bladder occupies almost the entire fetal abdomen.

if the pregnancy is not interrupted. Pregnancy termination is an option, but an autopsy is invaluable. A genetic syndrome like Meckel–Gruber may be associated with renal agenesis and has autosomal recessive inheritance, with a high risk of recurrence.

The other possibility is bladder outflow obstruction. The bladder is likely to be abnormally enlarged, almost filling the whole of the fetal abdomen. There may be evidence of ureteric and renal pelvic dilatation. Presence of fetal obstructive uropathy is a difficult challenge for management (Fig. 3.2). The possibility of introducing a vesicoamniotic shunt exists. However, pre-existing renal damage and/or lung hypoplasia cannot be reversed. Although fetal survival can be substantially improved, the long-term outcome is less encouraging. There is a high risk of end-stage renal failure requiring long-term dialysis or renal transplantation in the first few years of life. There also is a high risk of problems with voiding due to bladder dysfunction and catheter dependence. Additionally, there is a risk of bladder obstruction due to a cloacal abnormality, in which case, reconstruction of the external genitals (usually in females) may need to be done after birth. All these factors should be considered while planning management of such a case.

Severe Early Onset Fetal Growth Restriction

Severe early onset growth restriction is uncommon. It should be suspected when anhydramnios or severe oligohydramnios is seen, but there is no history of membrane rupture, and a normal fetal urinary bladder is visualised. The most common cause is severe placental insufficiency. Supporting evidence can be found in most cases. If an early dating scan has been carried out (thereby excluding wrong dates), the fetal size is often below the 5th centile. Uterine artery Doppler indices are likely to be abnormal. If the growth restriction is so severe as to lead to anhydramnios, there is often evidence of absent or reversed end diastolic flow in the umbilical artery, mild dilatation of the heart with abnormal ductus venosus Doppler and evidence of echogenic bowel due to ischemia. The placental echotexture is often abnormal, and the placenta could be enlarged, jelly-like or small with advanced maturity and placental echogenicities (Fig. 3.3).

In rare cases the fetal growth restriction is caused by primary fetal problems, such as a chromosomal abnormality. The amniotic fluid volume is more often normal, and other abnormalities may be seen on the scan.

The absence of amniotic fluid in placental insufficiency is not completely explained by the physiology of amniotic fluid dynamics. In experimental animal studies, fetal hypoxia was found to be associated with increased urine production rather than oliguria. Oligo/Anhydramnios seen in placental insufficiency may be due to increased absorption of the amniotic fluid across the fetal membranes overlying the placenta.

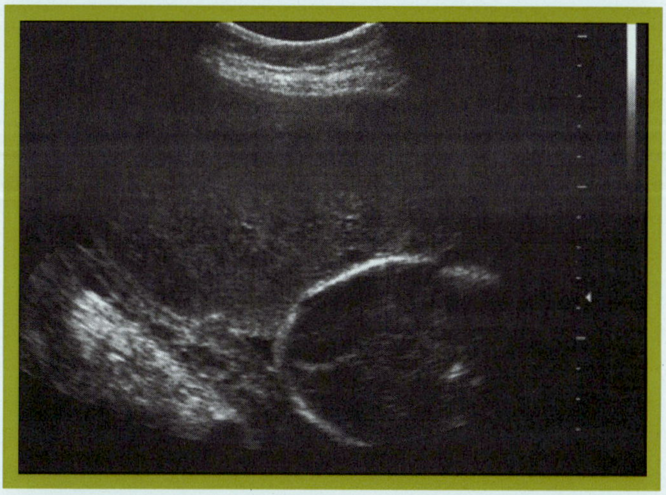

Figure 3.3: Abnormal placenta with early onset placental insufficiency; the placenta appears enlarged and heterogeneous in echotexture.

Management is dictated by the severity of growth restriction, gestational age and estimated fetal weight. The optimum method of monitoring such pregnancies is uncertain, and the two potential methods are fetal cardiotocography (preferably computerised) or ductus venosus Doppler indices. Delivery is usually not indicated unless the gestational age is at least 26 weeks and the estimated fetal weight 500 g. Antenatal neonatal consultations should be organised so that parents can participate in the decision for delivery. If neonatal intensive care unit beds are unavailable, an in utero transfer to a unit with a vacant bed is preferable to an ex utero transfer.

Further Reading

- Baschat A. 2004. Doppler application in the delivery timing of the preterm growth-restricted fetus: Another step in the right direction. *Ultrasound Obstet Gynecol* 23:111–18.
- Clark J, W Martin, T Divakaran, M Whittle, M Kilby and K Khan. 2003. Prenatal bladder drainage in the management of fetal lower urinary tract obstruction: A systematic review and meta-analysis. *Obstet Gynecol* 102:367–82.
- Freedman A, M Johnson, C Smith, R Gonzalez and M Evans. 1999. Long-term outcome in children after antenatal intervention for obstructive uropathies. *Lancet* 354:374–77.
- Major CA and JL Kitzmiller. 1990. Perinatal survival with expectant management of midtrimester rupture of membranes. *Am J Obstet Gynecol* 163:838–44.

CHAPTER 4

INCREASED AMNIOTIC FLUID VOLUME

Case: An ultrasound scan was requested on account of the fundal height measurement being above the expected. Normal fetal growth was confirmed. No major abnormalities were found. Increased amniotic fluid volume was reported. The cause was unexplained.

Increase in amniotic fluid volume is often referred to as polyhydramnios. There are several definitions for this entity but none are universally agreed upon. Two commonly used definitions are given below:

- Amniotic fluid index (AFI) above the 95th centile for gestation (often AFI >25 cm).
- Maximum vertical pocket of amniotic fluid measuring >8 cm.

Neither AFI nor maximum vertical pocket correlates with the actual amniotic fluid volume.

Causes

By the first definition, the prevalence of polyhydramnios is expected to be about 5%. Many of the polyhydramnios cases are apparently unexplained. The possible causes are given below:

Maternal diabetes in pregnancy: The association between poor maternal diabetes control and polyhydramnios is well-established. Polyhydramnios is thought to result from fetal polyuria. This is caused by fetal osmotic diuresis as a consequence of maternal and fetal hyperglycemia. Maternal blood glucose levels and maternal

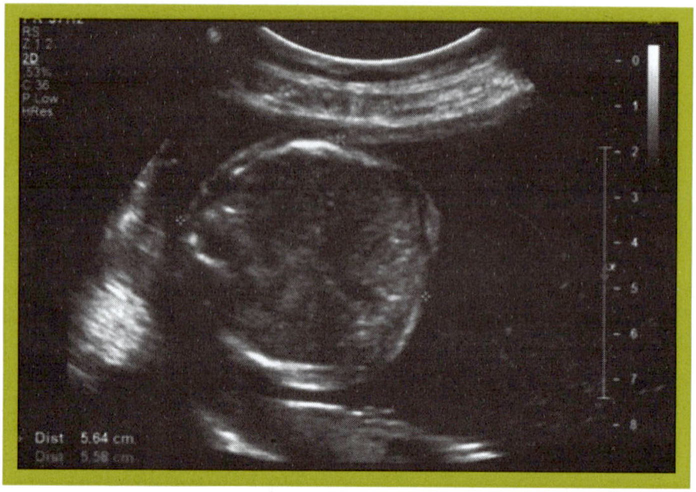

Figure 4.1: A case of suspected esophageal atresia; the stomach is not visualised and the amniotic fluid is excessive.

HbA1c are indicated in cases of polyhydramnios to exclude diabetes complicating the pregnancy.

Fetal abnormalities affecting fetal swallowing: Esophageal atresia is associated with a tracheoesophageal fistula (TOF) in a large proportion of cases. The fetal stomach can be filled by means of the alternate pathway, and polyhydramnios rarely develops. In a few cases, without a connection to the trachea the fetus is unable to swallow amniotic fluid. The fetal stomach is not visualised on persistent scanning and polyhydramnios develops after 26 weeks of gestation (Fig. 4.1).

The pediatric surgeon should be alerted, and delivery should take place at a centre with pediatric surgical facilities. Having said that, spontaneous preterm labour due to polyhydramnios is very common, and planned labour induction is very difficult to achieve.

Fetal duodenal atresia is rarely associated with a bypass and almost always progresses to severe polyhydramnios after 26–28 weeks. A double-bubble sign is characteristic due to atresia of the second part of the duodenum (Fig. 4.2). Congenital diaphragmatic hernia (CDH) often shows evidence of fetal stomach in the thorax and can lead to a mediastinal shift. Obstruction due to kinking can explain the polyhydramnios. Identification of polyhydramnios in cases of congenital diaphragmatic hernia is associated with a poorer prognosis.

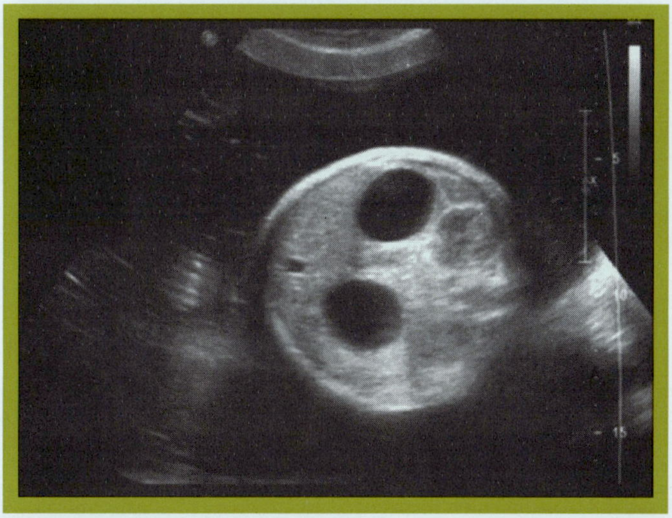

Figure 4.2: Fetus with duodenal atresia; note the typical double-bubble appearance and excess amniotic fluid volume.

Lethal skeletal dysplasia results in severe shortening of long bones and narrowing of the fetal thorax. The fetal lungs are unable to develop, and death is usually caused by pulmonary insufficiency (Fig. 4.3).

Polyhydramnios is caused by the inability of the fetus to swallow. Fetal akinesia leads to polyhydramnios. Severe polyhydramnios can also develop in a case of congenital myotonia.

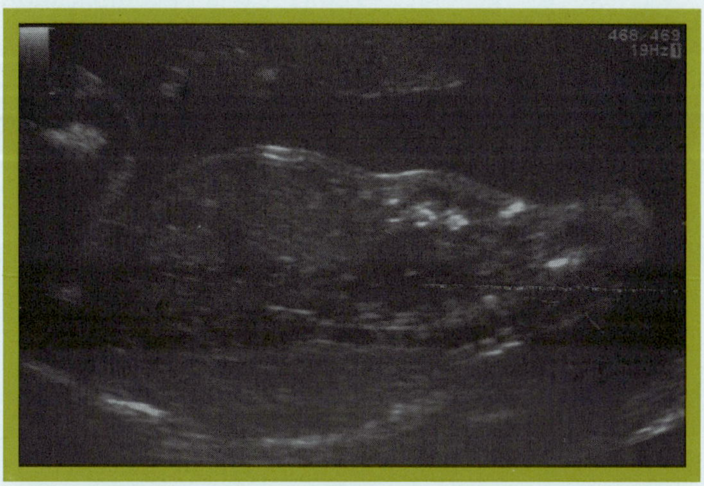

Figure 4.3: Fetus with lethal skeletal dysplasia; note the narrow thorax.

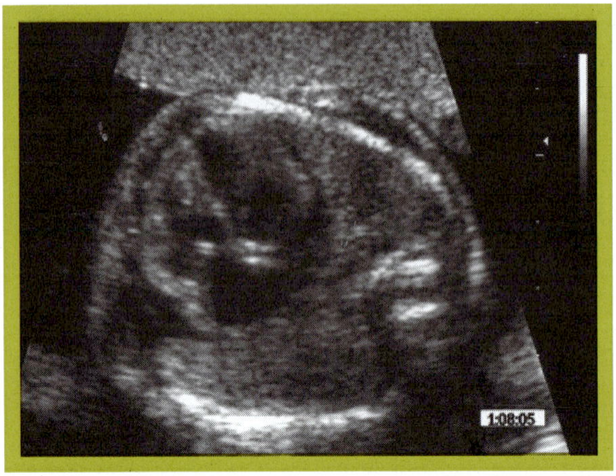

Figure 4.4: A fetus with parvovirus B19 infection; note the presence of pericardial effusion and mild enlargement of the heart.

Fetal cardiac failure: Accumulation of excess fluid in two or more serous cavities is defined as hydrops fetalis. Severe fetal anemia due to red cell isoimmunisation may lead to hydrops. However, with the advent of anti-D prophylaxis and screening for atypical antibodies at the booking visit, immune hydrops has become increasingly uncommon. Non-immune hydrops can develop because of a variety of reasons, and polyhydramnios is a very common accompanying feature. Figure 4.4 shows a fetus with severe fetal anemia due to fetal parvovirus B19 infection.

Placental chorioangiomas are seen on histology in approximately 1% of placentas. However, if the diameter is larger that 3–4 cm, pregnancy complications such as fetal anemia, fetal cardiac failure, hydrops and polyhydramnios may develop.

Figure 4.5 shows the typical ultrasound appearance of a placental chorioangioma. Fetal blood transfusion, amniodrainage and interstitial laser therapy are some of the treatment modalities used.

Multiple pregnancy and its complications: Polyhydramnios may develop in any variety of twin pregnancy (mono as well as dichorionic twins). Refer to *Chapter 2, Twin Gestation and Invasive Testing* and *Chapter 15, Twin-to-Twin Transfusion Syndrome* for details.

Management

Polyhydramnios is associated with increase in the risk of preterm delivery following spontaneous preterm labour. Logically, treatment of polyhydramnios should be

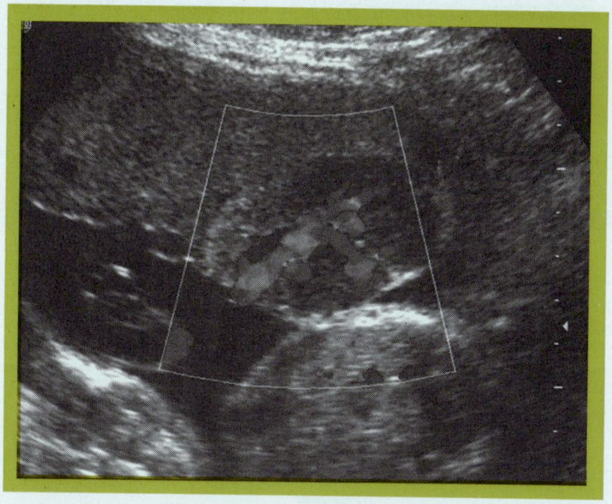

Figure 4.5: Placental chorioangioma seen on colour flow mapping

treatment of the cause. However, treatment of the cause is not always possible before birth (esophageal atresia). Polyhydramnios is associated with preterm labour and birth. A potential intervention is amnioreduction to bring down this risk. The rationale behind amnioreduction is to restore normal amniotic pressure by draining a large quantity of amniotic fluid volume, thereby reducing maternal discomfort, improving uteroplacental perfusion and prolonging pregnancy by limiting the risk of preterm labour and rupture of membranes. The procedure has a complication rate in terms of spontaneous premature rupture of membranes, abruptio placenta and chorioamnionitis regardless of the technique adopted. In a large study of amnioreduction procedures, the complication rate was relatively low at 3.1%.

Further Reading

- Leung WC, JM Jouannic, J Hyett, C Rodeck and E Jauniaux. 2004. Procedure-related complications of rapid amniodrainage in the treatment of polyhydramnios. *Ultrasound Obstet Gynecol* 23:154–58.
- Magann EF, SP Chauhan, PS Barrilleaux, NS Whitworth and JN Martin. 2000. Amniotic fluid index and single deepest pocket: Weak indicators of abnormal amniotic volumes. *Obstet Gynecol* 96:737–40.

Further Reading

- Many A, LM Hill, N Lazebnik and JG Martin. 1995. The association between polyhydramnios and preterm delivery. *Obstet Gynecol* 86:389–91.

CHAPTER 5

ECHOGENIC BOWEL

Case: A routine anomaly scan was performed at 22 weeks in a first pregnancy. The fetal measurements were within the reference range. However, the bowel was found to be hyper-echogenic in the scan. The parents were concerned about the possible implications.

Hyper-echogenicity of fetal bowel is a subjective finding. There is no objective definition for 'increased' echogenicity. If the echogenicity is as dense as the fetal bone, it is considered abnormal. However, echogenicity is influenced by the settings of the ultrasound equipment. The lack of an objective definition is one of the reasons why there is little consistency in the literature regarding its significance (Fig. 5.1).

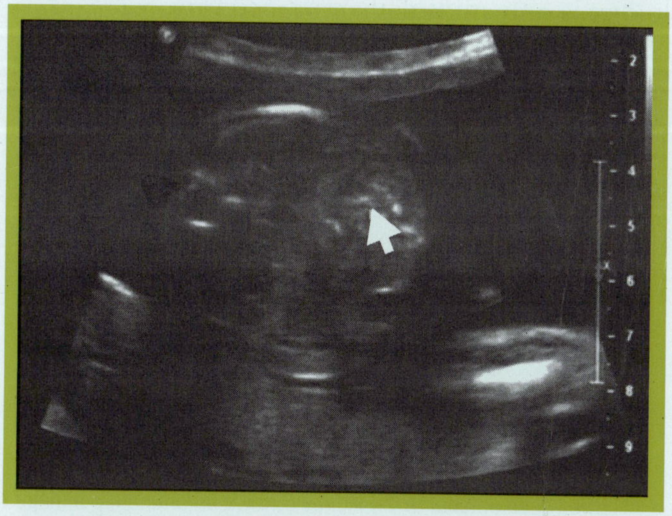

Figure 5.1: Echogenic bowel, indicated by the arrow

Hyper-echogenic bowel is often considered a soft marker for a chromosomal abnormality. Theoretically, the possibilities are as follows:

- Fetal growth restriction
- Chromosomal abnormalities
- Cystic fibrosis (CF)
- Meconium ileus
- Congenital viral infection (CMV)/Toxoplasmosis
- Intra-amniotic bleeding

Fetal Growth Restriction and Echogenic Bowel

The association of echogenic bowel and fetal growth restriction is well-known. The biometry is abnormal and often there is evidence of utero-placental insufficiency (refer to *Chapter 14, Suspected Fetal Growth Restriction*). Fetal echogenic bowel in IUGR fetuses is not associated with increased risk of neonatal necrotising enterocolitis.

Echogenic Bowel and Risk of Trisomies

The significance of echogenic bowel is modified by previous screenings. The risk of trisomies increases three times in a previously unscreened population. However, the finding loses significance in a pre-screened population, and the risk of aneuploidies is only minimally modified (Fig. 5.2).

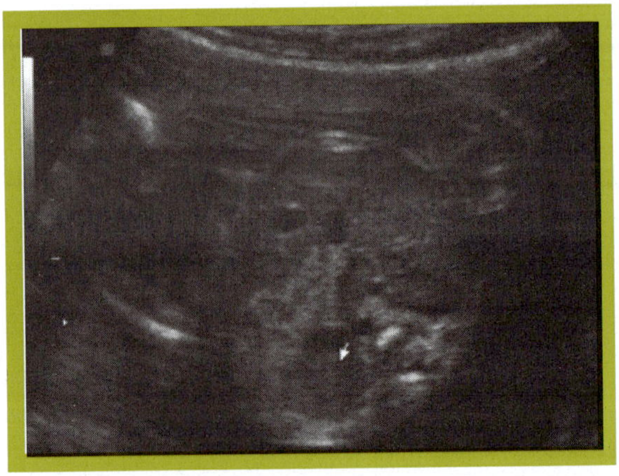

Figure 5.2: Echogenic bowel, seen anterior to the kidney (arrow); unfortunately, a major cardiac abnormality was also detected. The karyotype revealed Trisomy 13.

Cystic Fibrosis

Cystic fibrosis (CF) is an autosomal recessive genetic condition, associated with abnormally thick mucus secretion. The frequency of carrier status is 1:25 in Caucasians. However, carrier status is not associated with clinical symptoms. Only when the abnormal gene is inherited from both parents do clinical features appear. Several gene mutations have been identified—the commonest being the Δ F508 mutation. Carrier detection in prospective parents is difficult in view of the large number of mutations.

Prenatal diagnosis is possible if the specific mutation is identified. An invasive test such as CVS or amniocentesis is necessary. The risk of recurrence is one in four (25%) in the presence of an affected sibling.

Meconium Ileus

By definition, this is the obstruction of the intestine (ileus) due to an overly thick meconium. A leading underlying cause is cystic fibrosis.

Congenital Viral Infection

There are several reports establishing a link between congenital viral infections and echogenic fetal bowel. Fetal infection with cytomegalovirus (CMV) appears to have the strongest link. Infections with other viruses are uncommon, at least in the UK. Oligohydramnios, microcephaly and small for gestational age (SGA) are the other features of fetal CMV infection.

Intra-amniotic Bleeding

Intra-amniotic bleeding or stained amniotic fluid appears to be a relatively common cause of echogenic bowel, seen in 11% in one series of 215 cases. Interestingly, amniocentesis was performed in 196 (91%) cases, and the colour of the amniotic fluid was noted. It is well-established that fetal swallowing is an important mechanism in amniotic fluid dynamics. Swallowed blood can explain the echodensity in the fetal abdomen. A history of vaginal bleeding in early pregnancy is often present.

In a large study of 175 fetuses in 171 pregnancies over a seven-year period, fetal karyotyping, CF carrier detection and maternal infection serology were carried out. Five fetuses were affected with cystic fibrosis. Fetal karyotype was obtained in 139 cases, and autosomal trisomy was diagnosed in 5 cases (3.6%). In the study, 166 patients were tested for toxoplasmosis, and 111 for CMV. There were no cases of congenital toxoplasmosis. Maternal serologic and fetal pathologic evidence of CMV infection was seen in one case.

Further Reading

- Abdel-Fattah SA, A Bhat, S Illanes, JL Bartha and D Carrington. 2005. TORCH test for fetal medicine indications: Only CMV is necessary in the United Kingdom. *Prenat Diagn* 25:1028–31.
- Achiron R, R Mazkereth, R Orvieto, J Kuint, S Lipitz and Z Rotstein. 2002. Echogenic bowel in intrauterine growth restriction fetuses: Does this jeopardize the gut? *Obstet Gynecol* 100:120–25.
- Al-Kouatly HB, ST Chasen, J Streltzoff and FA Chervenak. 2001. The clinical significance of fetal echogenic bowel. *Am J Obstet Gynecol* 185:1035–38.
- Kesrouani AK, J Guibourdenche, F Muller et al. 2003. Etiology and outcome of fetal echogenic bowel. Ten years of experience. *Fetal Diagn Ther* 18:240–46.
- Nicolaides K. 2003. Screening for chromosomal defects. *Ultrasound Obstet Gynecol* 21:313–21.

CHAPTER 6

INTRACRANIAL CYSTS

Case: During a routine anomaly scan at 22 weeks, the ultrasonographer was alarmed to find an echo-poor structure in the fetal brain. There were concerns about the origin of the lesion and the possibility of brain damage and subsequent handicap.

Choroid Plexus Cyst

Choroid plexus cysts are perhaps the most common variety of intracranial cysts seen in the prenatal period and can be observed in 0.6–2.0% of all fetuses at 21–23 weeks in the general population (Fig. 6.1). It is probably a little higher at 11–14 weeks. These cysts were considered harmless when first described. However, an association between choroid plexus cysts and aneuploidy (particularly Trisomy 18) was soon identified. Many case series, particularly those containing older and high-risk women, reported

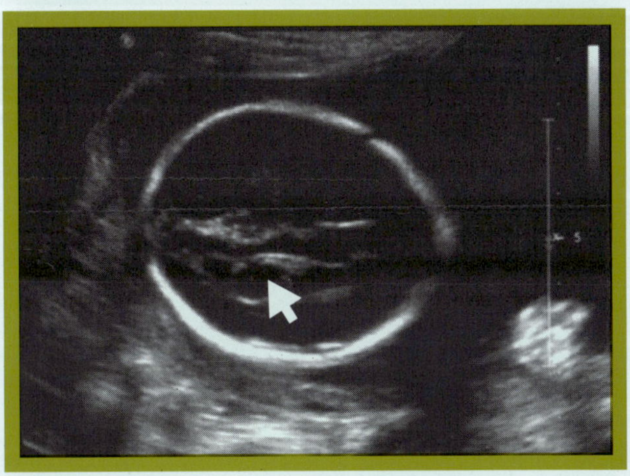

Figure 6.1: Transverse axial image of the fetal head showing a choroid plexus cyst (arrow)

a high risk of Trisomy 18 with choroid plexus cysts. These cysts are not associated with brain damage. They almost always disappear later in the pregnancy.

Posterior Fossa Cyst

Posterior fossa cysts include a variety of cysts and are discussed in *Chapter 11, Enlarged Cisterna Magna*. Frequent types of posterior fossa cysts are arachnoid, Blake's pouch and cysts associated with the Dandy–Walker malformation. A rare variety occurs as a result of a venous malformation and possible clot formation in the vein. Limited evidence suggests that the outlook is likely to be poor with a high risk of subsequent handicap. The cyst contents are somewhat echogenic on ultrasound evaluation. Ultrasound alone is not diagnostic, and other modalities such as MRI scan are required (Fig. 6.2).

Aneurysm of the vein of Galen is a rare malformation of the posterior cranial fossa. Vein of Galen is a cranial venous sinus that undergoes massive dilatation (Fig. 6.3).

Interhemispheric (Pseudo) Cyst

Interhemispheric cysts are seen in the midline and, by definition, between the two cerebral hemispheres. A large proportion of these are in fact not true cysts but collections of fluid between the hemispheres due to lack of a third ventricle roof. Often, associated deficiency of part or whole of the corpus callosum (agenesis of

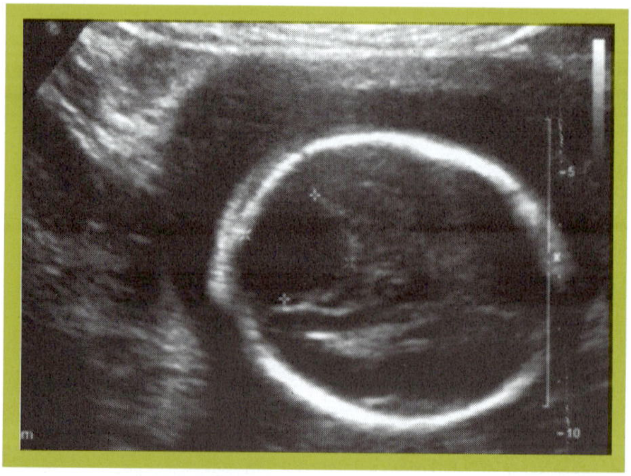

Figure 6.2: Transverse axial image through the fetal brain. Posterior fossa shows an echo-poor structure. If the venous malformation is thrombosed, no flow would be seen on colour flow mapping.

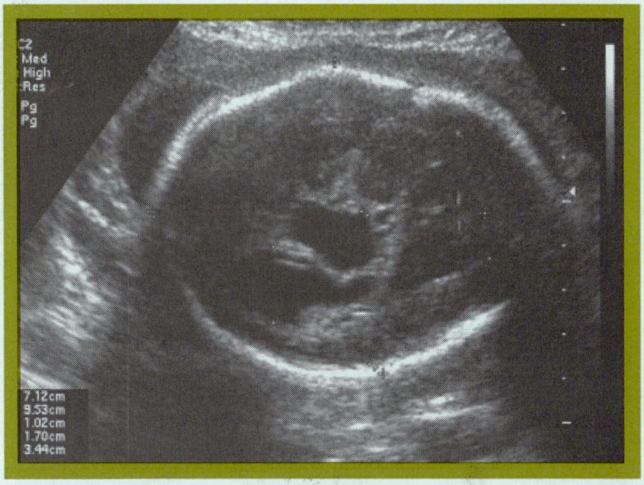

Figure 6.3: Transverse axial image showing aneurysm of vein of Galen

the corpus callosum or ACC) is seen. Many genetic syndromes are associated with ACC. In general, there is a high risk of neuro-developmental handicap associated with ACC, and the outlook is guarded. Ultrasound identification of the corpus callosum is possible, but difficult. Presence of ventriculomegaly, the tear-drop shape of the lateral ventricles and wider separation of the cavum should raise the suspicion of ACC. Fetal MRI helps greatly in the ascertainment of the presence of the corpus callosum (Figs 6.4 and 6.5).

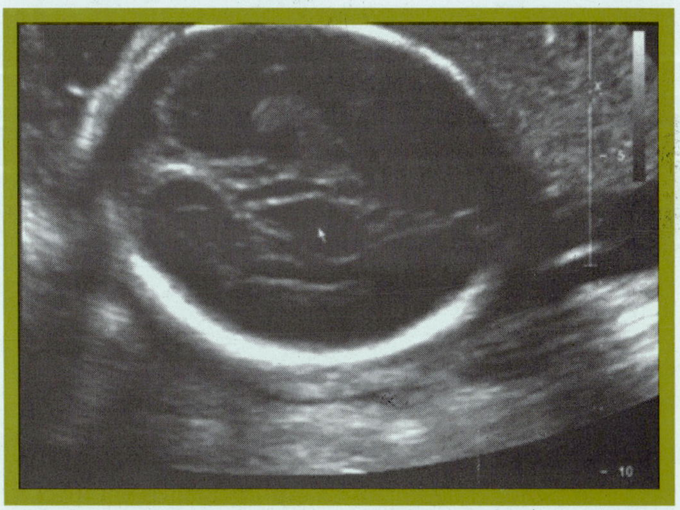

Figure 6.4: Interhemispheric 'cyst' associated with agenesis of the corpus callosum

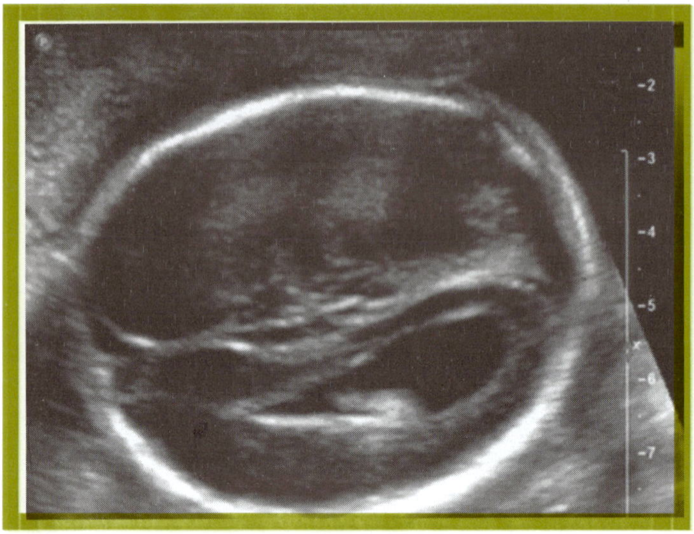

Figure 6.5: Typical 'tear-drop–shaped' lateral ventricle associated with agenesis of the corpus callosum

Arachnoid Cyst

Arachnoid cysts are collections of cerebrospinal fluid. They are benign, congenital, space occupying lesions of the central nervous system. The cysts are located within the layers of the arachnoid membrane and can communicate with the subarachnoid space. They are thought to be caused by an abnormal developmental process of the lepto-meninges. Small cysts are usually asymptomatic. Large cysts may lead to compression and hydrocephalus. Postnatally, they may cause seizures, headache and focal neurological signs. Size, gestational age at diagnosis and location of the cyst seem to influence the prognosis. Midline arachnoid cysts are often a consequence of ACC. The follow-up of 54 fetuses presenting with arachnoid cysts in the second and third trimesters reported good prognosis in 88% of persons, in terms of behaviour, neurological development and intelligence at 4 years. Some reports describe complete resolution of the cysts, and the cysts rarely progress postnatally (Fig. 6.6).

Work-up

Fetal MRI: Fetal MRI is of particular value in the prenatal evaluation of fetal CNS lesions. MRI does not involve ionising radiation and is safe in pregnancy. Fetal movement during the acquisition of MRI data will lead to deterioration of image quality. Hence 5 mg diazepam is often given to the mother to minimise

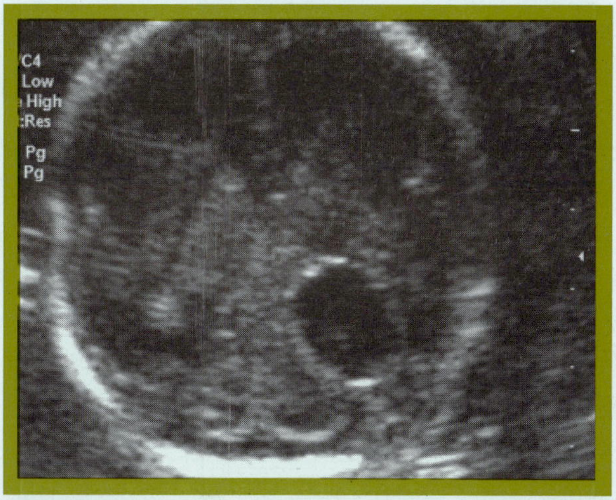

Figure 6.6: Fetal arachnoid cyst; note the paramedian location.

fetal activity. MRI provides important information not easily obtained by ultrasound scans. This includes surface sulcation, presence of the corpus callosum, differentiation of grey and white matter of the brain and presence of intracranial bleeding.

Karyotype: Karyotyping should be offered in cases of choroid plexus cysts and an additional high-risk factor. In the pre-screened population, the risk of a chromosomal abnormality is not increased. Fetuses with Trisomy 18 almost always have additional findings apart from choroid plexus cysts and should be assessed. Karyotyping should also be offered in cases of ACC, particularly when parents decide to continue the pregnancy.

Follow-up in Pregnancy

Where a choroid plexus cyst has been identified, a follow-up scan close to term (36 weeks) helps to exclude persistence and to relieve parental anxiety. In other cases where pregnancy has continued, a follow-up scan is helpful in assessing change in size and its effect on the brain if the size has increased. Very large cysts can lead to macrocephaly, thereby precluding vaginal birth. An elective cesarean section would be required. In intracranial cysts other than choroid plexus cysts, antenatal neurosurgical consultation would help address parental concerns and questions.

Further Reading

- Chitty LS, P Chudleigh, E Wright, S Campbell and M Pembrey. 1998. The significance of choroid plexus cysts in an unselected population: Results of a multicentre study. *Ultrasound Obstet Gynecol* 12:391–97.
- Fratelli N, AT Papageorghiou, F Prefumo, S Bakalis, T Homfray and B Thilaganathan. 2007. Outcome of prenatally diagnosed agenesis of the corpus callosum. *Prenat Diagn* 27:512–17.
- Pierre-Kahn A, P Hanlo, P Sonigo, D Parisot and RS McConnell. 2000. The contribution of prenatal diagnosis to the understanding of malformative intracranial cysts: State of the art. *Childs Nerv Syst* 16:619–26.

CHAPTER 7

MILD RENAL PELVIC DILATATION

Case: Routine anomaly scan was carried out in the second trimester of pregnancy. The operator noticed mild fullness of both renal pelvices. Amniotic fluid was normal. The possibility of an associated chromosomal abnormality was raised. The parents were very anxious.

There is no universally accepted definition for the term mild renal pelvic dilatation. Two commonly used definitions are:

- Anterioposterior (AP) renal pelvic dimension >5 mm before 20 weeks and >7 mm after 20 weeks
- AP renal pelvic dimension of 5–10 mm at 16 weeks

The prevalence of mild renal pelvic dilatation depends on the gestational age of the scan, definition used, fetal gender, fullness of the fetal bladder and

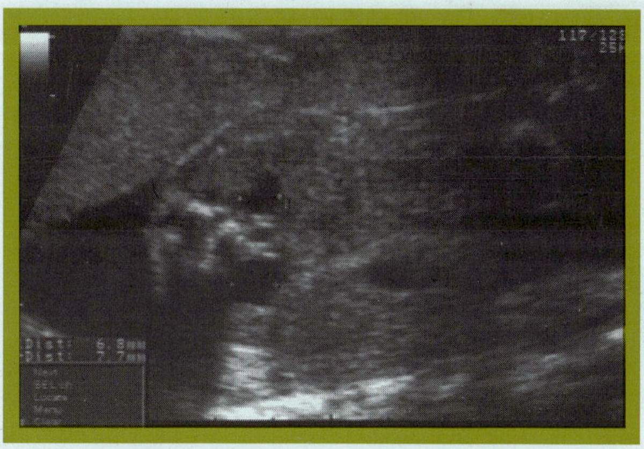

Figure 7.1: Bilateral renal pelvic dilatation

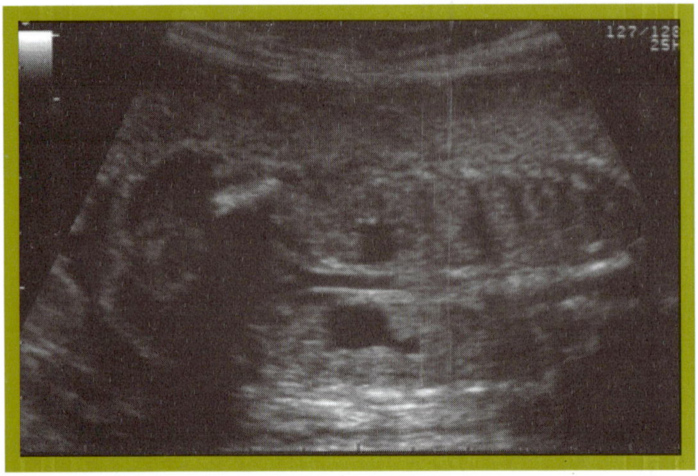

Figure 7.2: The same fetus seen on the longitudinal image

ultrasound equipment settings. The prevalence is 2–4% in an unselected population in most studies. It is twice as common in male fetuses, presumably due to the considerably longer length of the male urethra (Figs 7.1 and 7.2).

Kidneys and Bladder

Both the kidneys should be checked, as well as their echogenicity, which should be normal. Presence of increase in echogenicity and cortical cysts in the kidney is

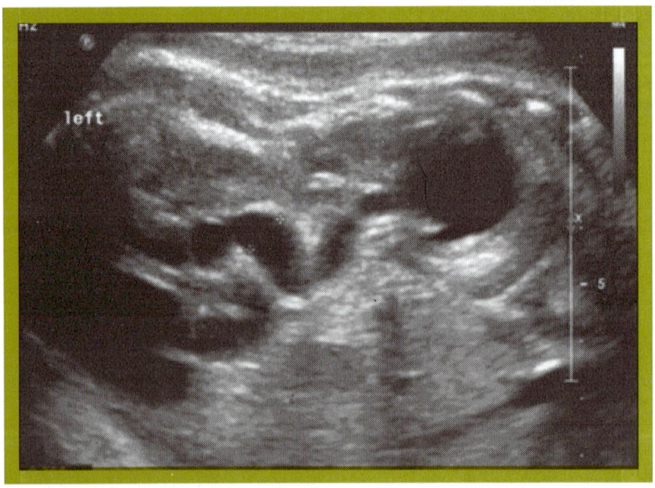

Figure 7.3: Dilated ureter on the left. The markers measure the diameter of the ureter. Normally, ureters should not be visible.

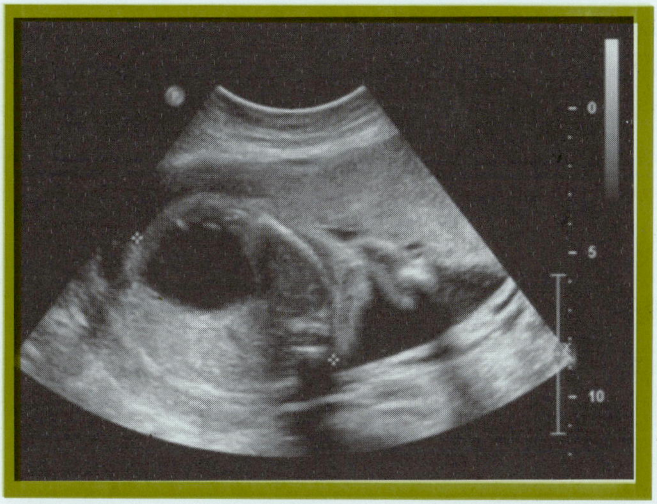

Figure 7.4: Large fetal urinary bladder seen in the second trimester. Normal amniotic fluid volume surrounding the fetus indicates preserved renal function.

associated with poor renal function. Ultrasound visualisation of the ureters must be attempted; normally, the ureters are not visible. Identification of the ureters raises the possibility of an obstruction or reflux (Fig. 7.3). Normal urinary bladder is visualised between the two umbilical arteries. Although there is no objective standard for normal bladder size, the bladder should be visible sometime during the period of scanning. Subjectively, the fetal bladder may be seen to be too big (Fig. 7.4).

The amniotic fluid quantity should also be checked. Amniotic fluid index (AFI) is an objective tool used to quantify the amniotic fluid volume. However, the sensitivity and specificity of AFI for the diagnosis of oligohydramnios is poor. Formal AFI measurement and measurement of the deepest vertical pool are equally satisfactory for identification of oligohydramnios and do not differ greatly from subjective assessment of adequacy of liquor volume.

Risk of Chromosomal Abnormality

Several publications have reported an association between mild renal pelvic dilatation and increased risk of trisomies. However, there are several problems with the risk estimation. Most studies do not take into account other risk factors such as maternal age or prior screening for Down syndrome when reporting their data. The likelihood ratio of isolated mild renal pelvic dilatation for the risk of Trisomy 21 was estimated at 1.5 by Pilu and Nicolaides. However, not all authors concur with this view. The widespread incorporation of Down syndrome screening in the first trimester has led to pre-selection. In a population previously screened with nuchal translucency, mild renal pelvic dilatation is not associated with an increase in the risk of Trisomy 21.

Care during Pregnancy

It is reasonable to repeat the scan at 32–34 weeks of pregnancy. Mild renal pelvic dilatation mid-pregnancy would show resolution of the dilatation at this time, which is reassuring. In some persons, the dilatation persists. In a small minority, the dilatation may worsen.

Impact on Postnatal Outcome

Several publications have reported that the renal pelvic dilatation seen mid-pregnancy resolves spontaneously before or after birth in a large majority of persons. The risk of postnatal surgery on the urinary tract is less than 5% in these fetuses.

Postnatal Care with Persistence of Renal Pelvic Dilation in the Third Trimester

Persons with renal pelvic dilatation mid-pregnancy that resolves at 32–34 weeks can be reassured, and no further renal follow-up is needed. Persons showing persistence or worsening of dilatation require follow-up. Dilatation of the urinary tract and resultant urinary stasis can lead to urinary tract infections and damage to renal function. It is a common policy to start prophylactic antibiotics for newborns who have been diagnosed with renal tract dilatation in utero. A postnatal renal ultrasound scan is usually organised; however, the renal system does not become fully functional until after the first week of life, and so the ultrasound scan should be delayed at least till then. If the ultrasound scan shows persistence of renal tract dilatation, antibiotics must be continued and follow-up organised with a pediatric surgeon with an interest in pediatric urology. Isotope scans of the renal tract and a micturating cystourethrogram (MCUG) are the next steps involved in the follow-up of these babies.

Further Reading

- Bhide A, MK Farrugia, S Sairam, SA Boddy and B Thilaganathan. 2005. The sensitivity of antenatal ultrasound for predicting renal tract surgery in early childhood. *Ultrasound Obstet Gynecol* 25:489–92.
- Chudleigh T. 2001. Mild pyelectasis. *Prenat Diagn* 21:936–41.
- Pilu G and KH Nicolaides. 1999. Features of chromosomal defects. In *Diagnosis of Fetal Abnormalities: The 18–23 Week Scan*. Parthenon Publishing: Carnforth, 99–104.
- Sairam S, A Al-Habib, S Sasson and B Thilaganathan. 2001. Natural history of fetal hydronephrosis diagnosed on mid-trimester ultrasound. *Ultrasound Obstet Gynecol* 17:191–96.

CHAPTER 8

INTRA-ABDOMINAL CYSTS

Case: An echo-poor lesion was seen in the fetal abdomen during a routine mid-pregnancy anomaly scan. The exact origin was unclear. No additional structural abnormalities were found.

Any echo-poor structure in the fetal abdomen, detected on prenatal ultrasound, is referred to as an intra-abdominal cyst.

Possible Origin

The exact origin of an intra-abdominal cyst is notoriously difficult to pinpoint on prenatal ultrasound scan. In most cases, it is not clinically relevant, as no intervention is necessary (Fig. 8.1). One of the difficulties in ascertainment is when

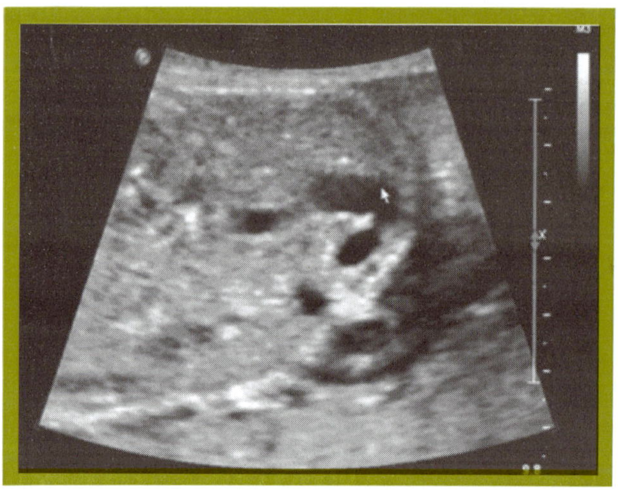

Figure 8.1: Ultrasound appearance of tubular intra-abdominal lesion (arrow); the diagnosis may remain unknown.

a cyst is identified on prenatal scan but the newborn is essentially asymptomatic, and an abdominal ultrasound scan is inconclusive. Further diagnostic workup, which is often invasive, unlike a simple ultrasound scan, is not justified in these cases, and the exact origin may remain uncertain. A definitive diagnosis is often not made until after the baby is born, and detection of an intra-abdominal cyst antenatally rarely alters obstetric management. The following is a list, which is by no means exhaustive, of some common causes:

Gastrointestinal tract

- *Duodenal atresia*: This is discussed in greater detail in *Chapter 4, Increased Amniotic Fluid Volume*. The classic ultrasound appearance is described as a 'double-bubble' sign. Polyhydramnios invariably appears after 26–28 weeks and most cases require amniodrainage. Spontaneous preterm delivery as a result of polyhydramnios or its treatment by amniodrainage is very common. The ultrasound features are typical, and prenatal diagnosis is fairly straightforward. It is unusual for duodenal atresia to be termed intra-abdominal cyst and not diagnosed as such.
- *Mid-gut obstruction*: Obstruction in the mid-gut may be a developmental defect or may develop secondary to conditions such as volvulus. Polyhdramnios is not a universal feature, particularly if it is a low small-

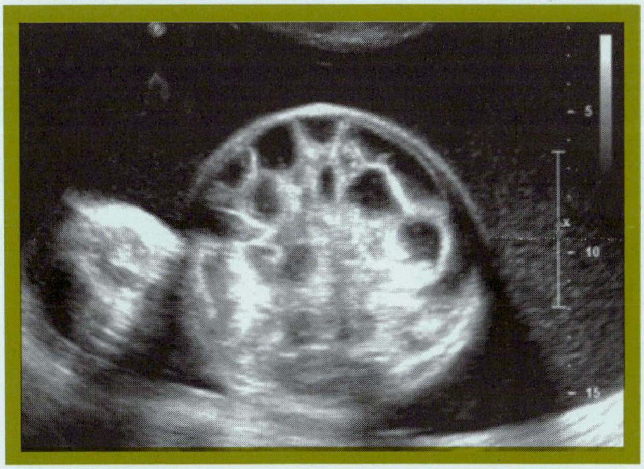

Figure 8.2: Ultrasound image of high-bowel obstruction; note the multiple bowel loops and excess amniotic fluid.

bowel obstruction. The part of the bowel proximal to the obstruction may become dilated, appearing as a 'cyst'. Typically, the 'cyst' margins are irregular, and it is often possible to demonstrate peristaltic movement. The dilated bowel loops are rarely single (Fig. 8.2).

- *Bowel duplication cyst*: This is a condition that occurs secondary to aberrant bowel development. It is benign if there is no bowel obstruction. The cyst is usually single, and polyhydramnios is not seen. Many cases are never confirmed after the baby is born as s/he may be clinically well and asymptomatic.
- *Choledochal cysts*: These are congenital anomalies of the bile ducts. They consist of cystic dilatations of the extrahepatic biliary tree, intrahepatic biliary radicles, or both. The ultrasound appearance of a double-bubble sign is similar to that in duodenal atresia, but polyhydramnios does not develop. Ultrasonically they occur in the upper abdomen and are indistinguishable from liver cysts (Fig. 8.3).
- *Mesenteric cysts*: These are benign lesions caused by fluid accumulation in the mesentery. No bowel obstruction is present. They are usually solitary. The newborn is likely to be asymptomatic.
- *Liver cysts*: Prenatal intervention is not required for these cysts. Regression without surgery is seen in most cases.

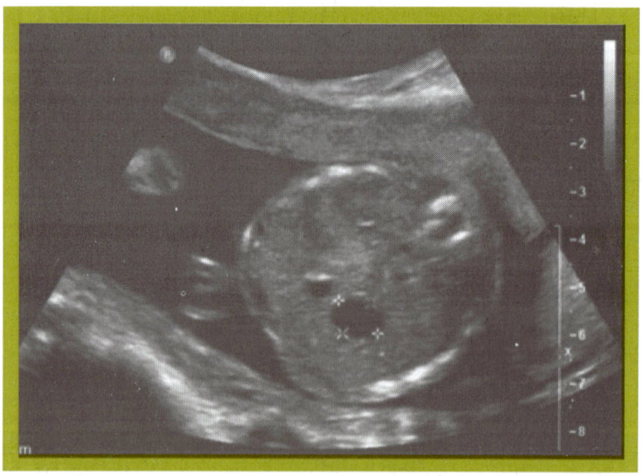

Figure 8.3: An echo-poor structure in close relation with the fetal liver. This could be a choledochal cyst or a liver cyst.

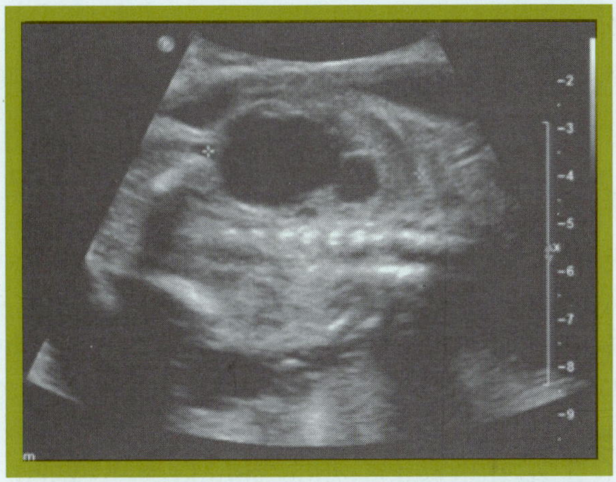

Figure 8.4: Ultrasound features of a multicystic dysplastic kidney; note the close proximity of the fetal spine.

Genito-urinary tract

- *Hydronephrosis/Cystic kidneys*: Detailed discussion of these conditions can be found in *Chapter 7, Mild Renal Pelvic Dilatation* and *Chapter 19, Obstructive Uropathy*. These are likely to be situated in close relation to the fetal spine (Fig. 8.4). The surrounding renal tissue can often be identified on ultrasound scan. Prenatal intervention is not indicated.
- *Fetal ovarian cysts:* These occur only in female fetuses. They are situated in close relation to the fetal bladder. Many disappear after birth (Fig. 8.5).

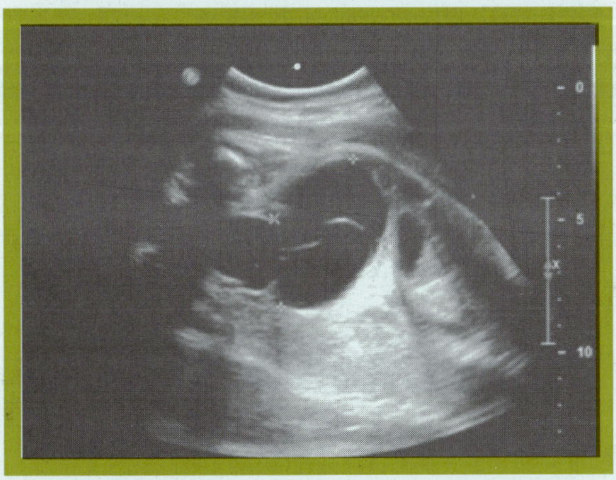

Figure 8.5: Ultrasound scan of fetal ovarian cyst (identified by the placement of cursors); note the close proximity to the bladder and the presence of septa.

Cysts of lymphatic origin

The origin is very difficult to identify prenatally. No flow is detected on colour flow mapping.

Care Plan for the Fetus

A detailed structural survey is indicated. Colour flow mapping is used to identify a vascular origin. The care plan is dependant on the probable origin of the cyst. If bowel obstruction is thought to be very likely, delivery should take place at a centre where pediatric surgical facilities are available. It is reasonable to arrange a follow-up scan in the third trimester to assess change in size. Neonatologists should be alerted at birth. Oral feeding should be started only after bowel obstruction has been excluded.

Post-delivery Care

An abdominal ultrasound scan is usually one of the first investigations carried out. Many cases can be managed conservatively. Further investigations are required if the newborn is symptomatic or if further complications are likely.

Further Reading

Heling KS, R Chaoui, F Kirchmair, S Stadie and R Bollmann. 2002. Fetal ovarian cysts: Prenatal diagnosis, management and postnatal outcome. *Ultrasound Obstet Gynecol* 20:47–50.

CHAPTER 9

POSITIVE UTERINE ARTERY DOPPLER SCREEN

Case: A 32-year-old woman underwent a routine anomaly scan at 22 weeks in her first pregnancy. Uterine arterial Doppler indices were obtained as part of the uterine artery Doppler screening programme. The indices were elevated on both sides, and there was bilateral notching in the flow velocity waveform.

Uterine artery was one of the first vessels to be assessed, initially using continuous wave Doppler and later, pulsed wave Doppler technology. Uterine artery blood flow was thought to reflect placentation, and abnormal uterine artery blood flow to reflect deficient trophoblastic invasion. Normal placental embedding converts high-resistance uterine blood flow into one of low resistance by the trophoblastic permeation of vascular media. Histopathological studies support this hypothesis.

Technique

Initially begun as a two-stage process (the first stage performed at 20–22 weeks and the second stage at 24–26 weeks), a single stage screening at 21–23 weeks is now preferred. It can conveniently be combined with the anomaly scan, a routine practice in many countries at around 20 weeks of pregnancy. Both transabdominal and transvaginal techniques have been described.

The transabdominal technique can be performed as part of the routine anomaly scan. Scanning is begun in each iliac fossa by tilting the transducer medially and caudally, till the iliac arteries are identified. Uterine arteries are identified as those that appear to cross the iliac arteries, using colour flow

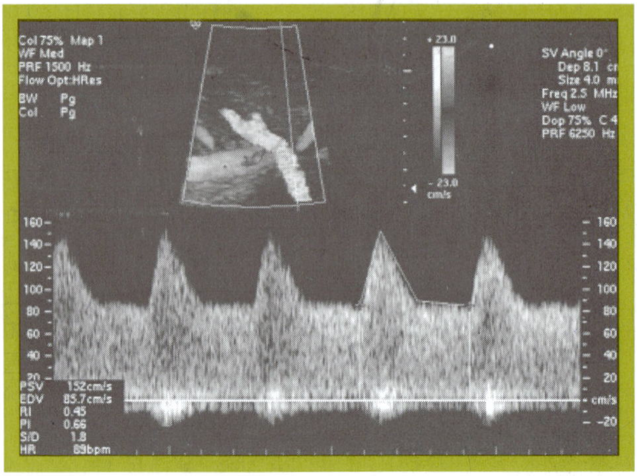

Figure 9.1: Normal uterine artery flow velocity waveform at 21–23 weeks' gestation; note the good diastolic flow and absence of diastolic notching.

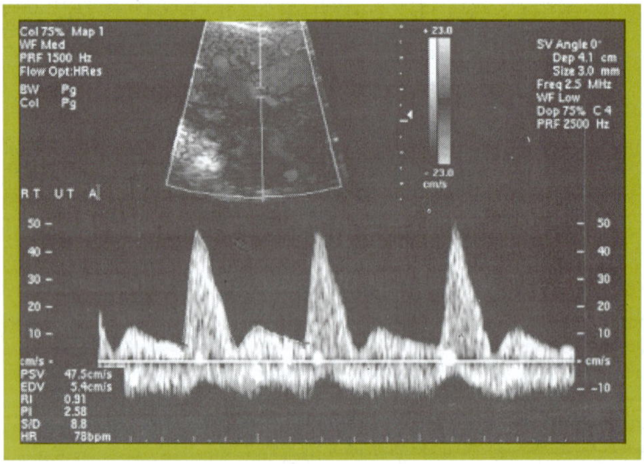

Figure 9.2: Abnormal uterine artery flow velocity waveform; note the deep diastolic notch and poor diastolic flow.

mapping. The sample volume is placed just distal to the apparent crossing of the uterine and iliac arteries. The typical flow velocity waveform of the uterine arteries is identified (Figs 9.1 and 9.2).

Positive Uterine Artery Doppler Screen

Early studies stressed the presence of a diastolic notch in the uterine artery Doppler flow velocity waveform to be abnormal. Later, it was realised that diastolic flow is also important. One study included cases with bilateral notching and mean RI >0.55 (50th centile) or unilateral notch with mean RI >0.65 (80th centile) as an abnormal uterine artery Doppler screen. A logical combination of these two has been the abandonment of the S/D ratio or RI, and incorporation of the pulsatility index (PI), which takes into account both diastolic flow and waveform 'pulsatility'. Currently, the 90th or 95th centiles are used as a 'cut-off'. A further complication is that there are two uterine arteries, and the waveforms are influenced by the laterality of the placenta. The most commonly used criterion is the use of mean PI cut-off. In the author's unit, a mean PI>1.25 (89th centile) was considered abnormal and yielded a screen-positive rate of 11%.

Uterine Artery Dopplers and Prediction of Pre-eclampsia

It is now widely accepted that a positive uterine artery Doppler screen correlates with the risk of development of preterm pre-eclampsia. The prevalence of pre-eclampsia (proteinuric hypertension) is about 2–4% in the population. Several screening studies using uterine artery Doppler for predicting pre-eclampsia and fetal growth restriction have been reported. A positive uterine artery Doppler screen is known to have a pooled likelihood ratio of 6.6 for the development of pre-eclampsia. Pre-eclampsia is a disease of primiparity. Bilateral notching in the uterine artery is more common in nulliparous than multiparous women. Pre-eclampsia is also more common in nulliparous women. Screening low-risk multiparous women with uterine arterial Dopplers for prediction of pre-eclampsia and fetal growth restriction is not thought to be effective, and this should be limited to nulliparous women.

The likelihood ratio of a positive uterine artery Doppler screen for high-risk women is lower that that for low-risk women, but due to the high prevalence, a positive screen increases the risk of developing pre-eclampsia (Table 9.1).

Uterine Artery Dopplers and Fetal Growth Restriction

The likelihood ratio of positive uterine artery Doppler screen for fetal growth restriction (as defined by the birth weight below the 10th centile) was 4.15 in a UK multicentre study. The sensitivity for detecting fetal growth restriction (as defined by birth weight below the 5th or 10th centile) is lower than that for pre-eclampsia.

Table 9.1: Performance of uterine artery Doppler screen (pulsatility index) for the detection of pre-eclampsia and fetal growth restriction

	Doppler Test Result	Prevalence %	Likelihood Ratio*	Post-test Probability (%)
		Clinically low-risk		
Pre-eclampsia	Positive	3	4.50	12.2
	Negative	3	0.64	1.8
Growth restriction	Positive	10	3.40	27.4
	Negative	10	0.87	8.8
		Clinically high-risk		
Pre-eclampsia	Positive	15	1.80	24.1
	Negative	15	0.78	12.0
Growth restriction	Positive	28	2.30	47.0
	Negative	28	0.56	17.9

*Likelihood ratios based on Cnossen et al 2008.

Uterine Artery Doppler and Risk of Antepartum Stillbirth

A recent study reported a large number of cases who had undergone uterine artery Doppler assessment mid-pregnancy. Stillbirth was considered 'placental' when there was evidence of placental abruption or when the mother had severe pre-eclampsia. In the absence of a direct cause, stillbirths were classified as unexplained. The risk of placental stillbirth increased among women with a mean PI in the top decile (adjusted HR was 5.5). The association with unexplained stillbirth was weaker (adjusted hazard ratio [HR] was 2.5). Abnormal uterine artery Doppler was better at predicting preterm stillbirth.

Further Reading

- Aquilina J, A Barnett, O Thompson and K Harrington. 2000. Comprehensive analysis of uterine artery flow velocity waveforms for the prediction of pre-eclampsia. *Ultrasound Obstet Gynecol* 16:163–70.

Further Reading

- Coomarasamy A, D Braunholtz, F Song, R Taylor and KS Khan. 2003. Individualising use of aspirin to prevent pre-eclampsia: A framework for clinical decision making. *Br J Obstet Gynaecol*110:882–88.
- Papageorghiu A, C Yu, R Bindra, G Pandis and KH Nicolaides. 2001. Multicenter screening for pre-eclampsia and fetal growth restriction by transvaginal uterine artery Doppler at 23 weeks of gestation. *Ultrasound Obstet Gynecol* 18:441–49.
- Smith G, C Yu, A Papageorghiou, A Cacho and K Nicolaides. 2007. Maternal uterine artery doppler flow velocimetry and the risk of stillbirth. *Obstet Gynecol* 109:144–51.
- Cnossen JS, RK Morris, G Riet, BW Mol, JA van der Post, A Coomarasamy, AH Zwinderman, SC Robson, PJ Bindels, J Kleijnen and KS Khan. 2008. Use of uterine artery Doppler ultrasonography to predict pre-eclampsia and intrauterine growth restriction: A systematic review and bivariable meta-analysis. *CMAJ* 178:701-11.

CHAPTER 10

VENTRICULOMEGALY

Case: An anomaly scan was carried out mid-pregnancy. The fetus was normally grown. The measurement of the lateral ventricles was 11 mm on repeated measurement. No other obvious malformation was seen on the scan. The parents were concerned about the possibility of mental retardation in the baby.

The posterior horn of the lateral ventricles is relatively easy to measure in the same section as that used to measure the biparietal diameter (BPD) and head circumference (HC). The technique used to measure the lateral ventricles has been standardised. It is recommended that the lateral ventricle be measured from inner wall to inner wall at the level of the glomus of the choroid plexus. Both the lateral ventricles should be scanned, although formal measurement on both sides is not required. In general, it is easier to make a measurement on the hemisphere distal to the probe, as near reverberation artifacts often obscure the measurement from the hemisphere closer to the probe. Tilting of the probe to one side may be useful in visualising the proximal lateral ventricle.

Definition

The ratio of the posterior horn to the cerebral hemisphere (Vp/H ratio) was originally employed to define normality. However, an absolute measurement has increasingly been reported in the literature. The lateral ventricles should normally measure up to 10 mm. Any measurement above this is considered to be out of the reference range. It is often classified, depending on the width of the posterior horn, as mild (10–12 mm), moderate (12.1–14.9 mm) or severe (>15 mm).

Unilateral Versus Bilateral Ventriculomegaly

Literature suggests that unilateral ventriculomegaly runs a benign course by and large, and the outlook is likely to be excellent. Bilateral ventriculomegaly, on the other hand, carries a more cautious prognosis. To some extent, the likelihood of an underlying sinister cause is dependant on the actual measurement. However, the prognosis depends on the underlying cause rather than the actual measurement.

Possibilities

Chromosomal abnormality: All the commonly seen trisomies (21, 18 and 13) are associated with ventriculomegaly, but it is likely to be mild rather than severe. In addition, fetuses with triploidy may also have ventriculomegaly. Other markers are often present. A congenital heart abnormality is present in over 95% of fetuses with Trisomy 18 or 13. This figure is 50% with Trisomy 21.

Brain abnormalities: Fetuses with spina bifida exhibit typical skull signs (lemon-shaped skull and banana-shaped cerebellum). These are reliable signs of an open spinal defect. However, the skull signs may disappear in late pregnancy, beyond 26–28 weeks (Figs 10.1, 10.2 and 10.3).

Neuronal migration disorders can lead to a wide spectrum of abnormalities that includes mild ventriculomegaly. Agenesis of the corpus callosum (ACC) is a rare abnormality and can lead to a typical tear-drop–shaped lateral ventricle.

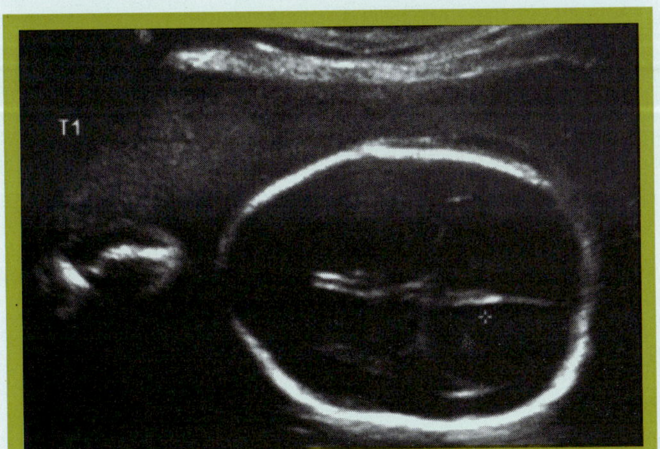

Figure 10.1: Lemon-shaped head in a case of spina bifida; note the presence of ventriculomegaly.

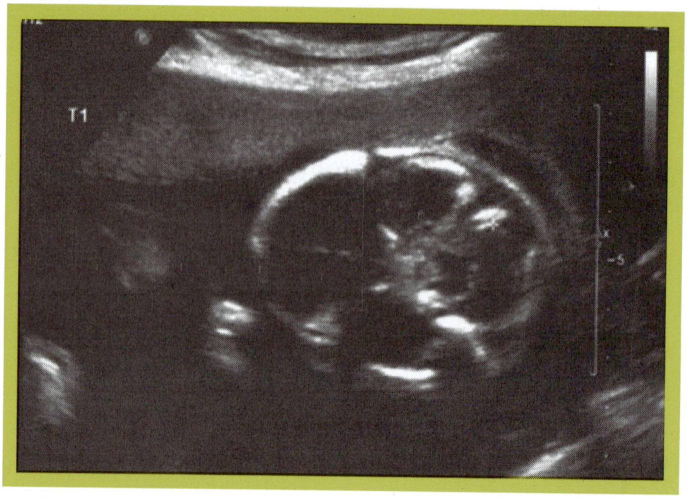

Figure 10.2: Banana-shaped cerebellum in a case of spina bifida; note that the cisterna magna cannot be measured as it is absent.

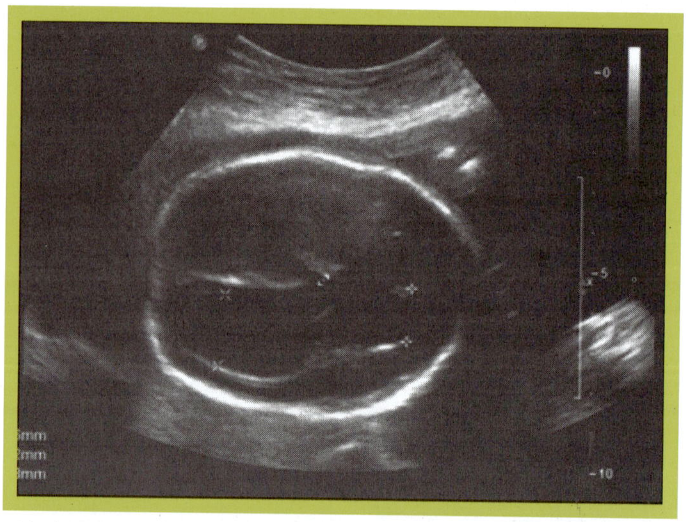

Figure 10.3: Ventriculomegaly in a case of aqueductal stenosis; the ventricular width measures 17.6 mm.

An interhemispheric 'pseudocyst' may also be seen (Fig. 10.4). More than half the cases have other malformations. Several genetic syndromes are associated with ACC. The outlook is guarded even if other abnormalities are not seen.

The cause of aqueductal stenosis is unknown in most cases. The ventriculomegaly is often severe and progressive, resulting in a large head circumference.

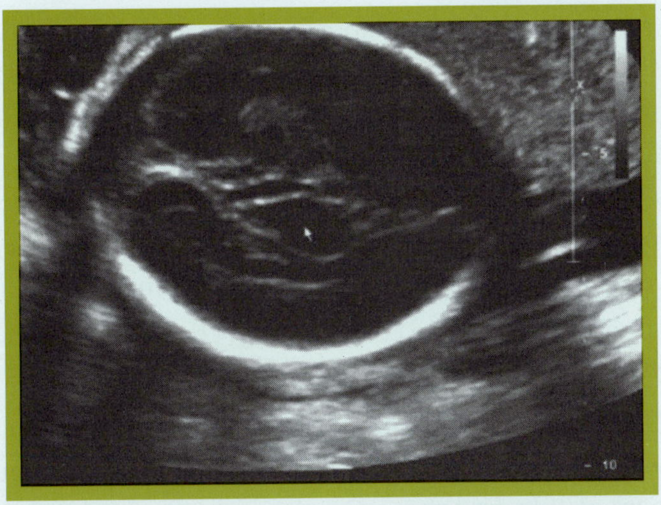

Figure 10.4: Interhemispheric cyst (arrow) in a case of agenesis of corpus callosum (ACC)

Viral infections: Congenital infection with cytomegalovirus or toxoplasmosis can lead to bilateral ventriculomegaly. The enlargement is rarely severe. Maternal primary CMV infection in pregnancy is associated with a 1 in 3 chance of fetal infection. With toxoplasma, the risk of fetal infection following primary maternal infection is gestation-related, being lower in early pregnancy and higher later.

Normal variant: The limit of 10 mm for defining normality is based on statistics, and corresponds to the 95th centile. By definition, 5% of normal fetuses will be above this limit. The more above the 10 mm cut-off the measurements are, the higher the chance that they are not a variation of the normal. Diagnosis of a normal variant is a diagnosis of exclusion. Lateral ventricular measurements are larger in male fetuses.

Investigations

The following investigations should be considered:

- Amniocentesis for karyotype should be considered if there are features of chromosomal abnormality or if the parents seek assurance of absence of a chromosomal abnormality. The amniotic fluid left after centrifugation and separating fetal cells should be saved, in case a congenital infection is suspected (instructions should be given to the cytogenetics laboratory).

- Maternal serology can be used to exclude congenital infection. If primary CMV or toxoplasma infection in pregnancy can be excluded, it is safe to eliminate infection as a possible cause of ventriculomegaly. Amniotic fluid testing using molecular biology techniques may be carried out to check for fetal infection if primary maternal infection in pregnancy is suspected. CMV or toxoplasma antigen testing can be carried out on the amniotic fluid after fetal cells have been separated for karyotyping.
- Fetal blood sampling may be considered to check the chromosomes, as it is quicker to obtain a full karyotype from leucocytes in the fetal blood.
- Fetal MRI is better at revealing the presence and normality of some brain structures such as sulci on the cerebral cortex or corpus callosum. Development of sulci and gyri on the brain surface changes with gestational age. Considerable experience is required to interpret MRI images. MRI and ultrasound scans are complimentary.

Prognosis

The prognosis of ventriculomegaly depends on the cause. The outlook is likely to be poor with chromosomal abnormalities and structural brain problems such as ACC or neuronal migration disorders. If fetal infection is proven, ultrasound evidence of ventriculomegaly usually means that the fetus has been affected, and other problems should be expected. Intelligence is expected to be normal in cases of spina bifida. Any problems related to intelligence are linked to CNS infection following a shunt procedure.

The outlook for unilateral mild ventriculomegaly is excellent. Chromosomal abnormalities are not associated. With bilateral mild ventriculomegaly, the outlook is generally good in the absence of an identifiable cause. In cases with ventricular width of up to 12 mm, 7–10% of babies showed developmental delay.

Further Reading

- Gaglioti P, D Danelon, S Bontempo, M Mombro, S Cardaropolli and T Todros. 2005. Fetal cerebral ventriculomegaly: Outcome in 176 cases. *Ultrasound Obstet Gynecol* 25: 372–77.

Further Reading

- Pilu G, P Falco, S Gabrielli, A Perolo, F Sandri and L Bovicelli. 1999. The clinical significance of fetal isolated cerebral borderline ventriculomegaly: Report of 31 cases and review of the literature. *Ultrasound Obstet Gynecol* 14: 320–26.
- Whitby E, M Paley, A Sprigg, S Rutter, N Davies, I Wilkinson and P Griffiths. 2004. Comparison of ultrasound and magnetic resonance imaging in 100 singleton pregnancies with suspected brain abnormalities. *Br J Obstet Gynaecol* 111:784–92.

CHAPTER 11

ENLARGED CISTERNA MAGNA

Case: During a routine anomaly scan carried out at 22 weeks, the size of the cisterna magna was found to be 10 mm. No other structural anomalies were seen. The sonographer was concerned about the possible implications of this finding.

Evaluation and Normal Anatomy of Cisterna Magna

The technique of imaging the fetal cerebellum and the cisterna magna has been standardised and published by the International Society of Ultrasound in Obstetrics and Gynecology (ISUOG). This plane is obtained at a slightly lower level than that of the transventricular plane and with a slight posterior tilting, and includes visualisation of the frontal horns of the lateral ventricles, cavum septum pelucidum (CSP), thalami, cerebellum and cisterna magna. The cisterna magna is the fluid-filled space posterior to the cerebellum. It contains thin septations, which are normal (Fig. 11.1).

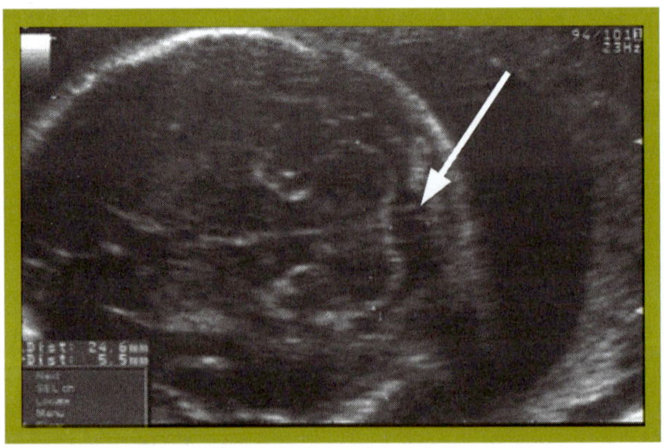

Figure 11.1: Normal posterior fossa; the septations are marked with an arrow.

In the second half of pregnancy, the depth of the cisterna magna is stable and should measure 2–10 mm. Early in gestation, the cerebellar vermis does not completely cover the fourth ventricle, and this may give a false impression of a vermian defect. Beyond 20 weeks, it should raise the suspicion of a cerebellar abnormality.

Nomenclature

Abnormalities of the cisterna magna with or without posterior fossa cysts were variously described as Dandy–Walker syndrome, Dandy–Walker spectrum or Dandy–Walker variant. Now it is recognised that this is not a single disorder, but a collection of distinct disorders with varying prognosis. The term 'Dandy–Walker syndrome' is best discarded, and the actual structural abnormality described.

Cerebellar Abnormality

Deficiency of the cerebellar vermis can produce the appearance of enlarged cisterna magna in the ultrasound scan (Figs 11.2, 11.3 and 11.4).

Cerebellar abnormalities on ultrasound scan must be assessed carefully. Unfortunately, the natural history of this disorder is modified by intervention. A large majority of prospective parents choose pregnancy termination when faced with a prenatal diagnosis of a probable brain abnormality. The older literature about this condition has a mixture of heterogeneous disorders grouped under the name

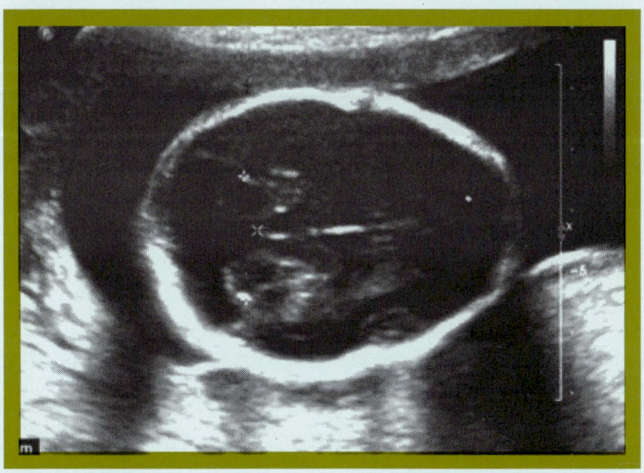

Figure 11.2: Complete agenesis of the cerebellar vermis; note the widely separated cerebellar hemispheres.

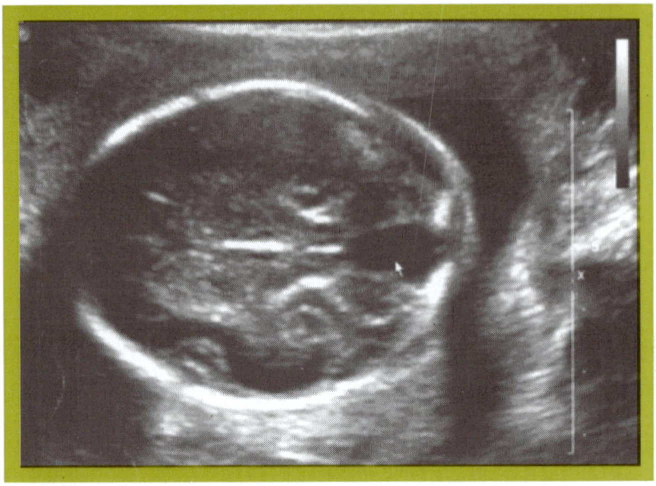

Figure 11.3: Ultrasound scan showing wide separation of cerebellar hemispheres (arrow) leading to enlarged cisterna magna

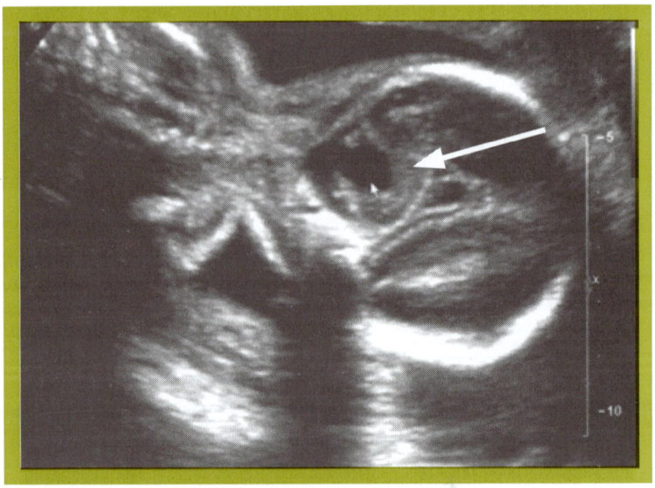

Figure 11.4: Same fetus as seen in Fig. 11.3; note that part of the cerebellar vermis is still present in the midline (broad arrow).

Dandy–Walker syndrome. Despite these problems, there is a >80% risk of long-term neuro-developmental handicap with prenatal diagnosis of this condition.

The separation of the cerebellar hemispheres can sometimes be visualised because of posterior and inferior rotation of the hemispheres, so that they appear to be hanging down. A scan plane that is too inferior can produce a false ultrasound appearance of partial deficiency.

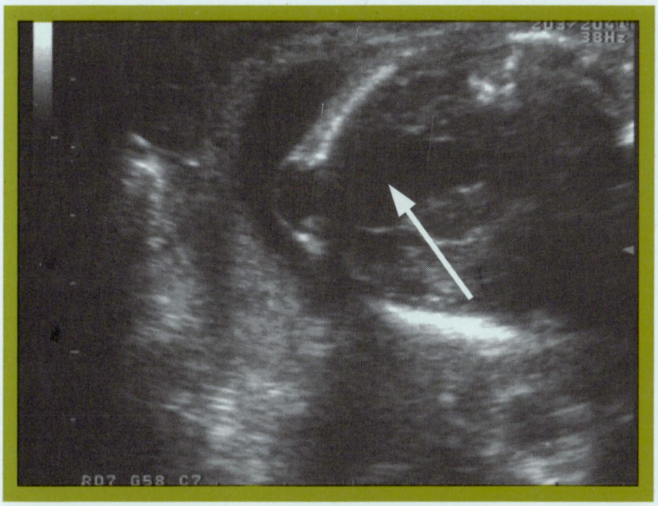

Figure 11.5: Ultrasound scan showing a cyst in the posterior fossa (arrow), and a deficiency in the occipital bone (encephalocele). The outlook is very guarded.

Cyst in the Posterior Fossa

A cyst in the posterior cranial fossa was previously included in the Dandy–Walker spectrum. It may be associated with a cerebellar abnormality, an abnormality of the skull table or a combination of both (Fig. 11. 5). Normal septations in the posterior fossa (Fig. 11.1) are in the midline and should not be interpreted as presence of a cyst.

Isolated Enlargement of Cisterna Magna

This used to be referred to as Dandy–Walker variant. An isolated enlargement of the cisterna magna without an underlying cerebellar abnormality is a benign finding. One should be careful not to angle the probe too far back and too low. This may lead to an erroneous finding of cisterna magna enlargement.

Genetic Syndromes

Joubert syndrome: This is a clinically and genetically heterogeneous group of disorders characterised by hypoplasia of the cerebellar vermis, with the neuroradiological 'molar tooth' sign and accompanying neurological symptoms, including dysregulation of breathing pattern and developmental delay.

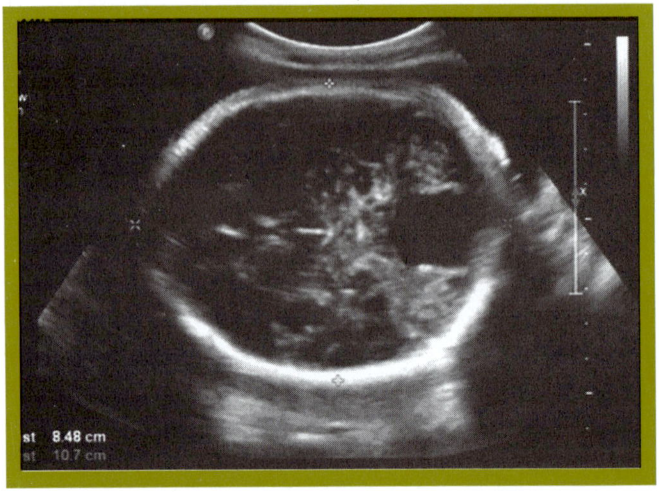

Figure 11.6: Antenatal ultrasound scan of Joubert syndrome

Figure 11.6 shows an ultrasound image of a fetus subsequently diagnosed with Joubert syndrome.

Meckel–Gruber syndrome/Meckel syndrome: Meckel syndrome is an autosomal recessive disorder characterised by a combination of renal cysts and variably associated features including developmental anomalies of the central nervous system (typically encephalocele), hepatic ductal dysplasia and cysts, and polydactyly. Although a variety of malformations have been observed, a frequent and particularly memorable combination is a sloping forehead, posterior encephalocele, polydactyly and polycystic kidneys. The recurrence risk is one in four.

Further Reading

- Aletebi F and KFK Fung. 1999. Neurodevelopmental outcome after antenatal diagnosis of posterior fossa abnormalities. *J Ultrasound Med* 18:683–89.
- International Society of Ultrasound in Obstetrics & Gynecology Education Committee. 2007. Sonographic examination of the fetal central nervous system: Guidelines for performing the 'basic examination' and the 'fetal neurosonogram'. *Ultrasound Obstet Gynecol* 29:109–16.

Further Reading

- Zalel Y, Y Gilboa, L Gabis, L Ben-Sira, C Hoffman, Y Wiener and R Achiron. 2006. Rotation of the vermis as a cause of enlarged cisterna magna on prenatal imaging. *Ultrasound Obstet Gynecol* 27:490–93.

CHAPTER 12

SHORTENING OF LONG BONES

Case: An anomaly scan was carried out mid-trimester in an uncomplicated pregnancy. No major structural defect was found. However, the femur length (FL) was found to be below the 5th centile on several measurement attempts. The possibility of skeletal dysplasia was raised.

When faced with shortening of the femur length, other long bones (humerus, forearm and leg bones) should be measured.

Possible Causes of Femur Length Below the 5th Centile

Problems with pregnancy dating

If the pregnancy has been dated incorrectly, fetal measurements may not be within the normal range. Pregnancies are best dated based on crown–rump length (CRL), obtained at 10–14 weeks. It is a national recommendation in many countries to date the pregnancy on CRL even if the menstrual dates are reliably known. If the pregnancy results from in vitro fertilisation, it should be dated from the day of the in vitro fertilisation (not the day of embryo transfer) rather than on CRL. If information about an early pregnancy scan is unknown, the pregnancy can be dated on the head circumference or transverse cerebellar diameter (TCD). The dating on fetal biometry is valid till 24 weeks.

In general, the earlier the pregnancy is dated the more reliable it is. A pregnancy cannot be reliably dated after 24 weeks. If a problem with dating the pregnancy is suspected, it is likely that all the fetal measurements (rather than only the femur length) will be out of sync with the gestational age reference range. After 24 weeks, pregnancy cannot be reliably dated, and a repeat scan in 2–4 weeks' time to look for interval growth may be the only option to confirm a dating error. Despite national recommendations, it is not uncommon to come across cases where menstrual dates rather than CRL was used for dating, and a situation similar to the one described above being encountered.

Constitutionally small fetus

Construction of the reference range is based on the statistical definition of 'normal'. About 5% of apparently normal and healthy fetuses are expected to show measurements below the 5th centile. All the measurements of a constitutionally small fetus are likely to be below the reference range, not just the femur length. The parents (particularly the mother) are likely to be of small build. It is important to use reference ranges derived from a multi-ethnic population. In general, fetal biometry matches maternal habitus more closely than paternal. The other differential diagnosis is fetal growth restriction. (Refer to *Chapter 14, Suspected Fetal Growth Restriction* for details).

Trisomy 21 (Down syndrome)

Individuals with Down syndrome often have short stature. It is not surprising to find an association with femur length below the 5th centile and Down syndrome. However, the association is not very strong, and the likelihood ratio is only 1.5. The humerus may be even shorter in fetuses with Trisomy 21. First trimester NT is likely to be increased in these cases. Approximately half the fetuses are likely to show evidence of a congenital heart abnormality such as atrio-ventricular septal defect. Routine screening for Trisomy 21 is now a common practice in many developed countries. The significance of a short femur is greatly reduced in populations that have undergone prior screening for Trisomy 21.

Focal femoral dysplasia

This is a heterogeneous condition in which one femur is short. If both are affected, they may be dissimilar in length. Differentiation from genetic skeletal dysplasia is difficult. However, isolated affliction with normality of other long bones is highly suggestive of this diagnosis. The babies usually need corrective surgery later.

Intrauterine growth restriction

Refer to *Chapter 14, Suspected Fetal Growth Restriction* for details.

Fetal skeletal dysplasia

Fetal skeletal dysplasia is not a single disorder, but a group of disorders that may lead to varying degrees of shortening of the small bones. A large study reported a crude prevalence rate of 2.3/10,000 at birth. However, several indications of under-registration suggest that the real value is about twice that observed. A family history of a 'bone problem' may indicate the possibility of skeletal dysplasia. However, many are new mutations, and no significant family history would be available.

From the point of view of clinical management, skeletal dysplasias can be broadly divided into two groups: lethal and non-lethal.

Lethal skeletal dysplasias: These exhibit severe shortening of the long bones. The length is below the 3rd (often below the 1st) centile for gestation. The fetal chest is narrow, and the fetal heart appears to fill a large part of the thorax on the four-chamber view (apparent cardiomegaly). This can be confirmed by measuring the cardiothoracic ratio (ratio of cardiac circumference to chest circumference in the 'transverse four-chamber' heart view) and comparing this ratio to the reference range.

Narrowing of the chest leads to lung hypoplasia, and this causes neonatal death due to respiratory insufficiency at birth. Significant narrowing of the chest often leads to development of polyhydramnios after 26 weeks due to interference

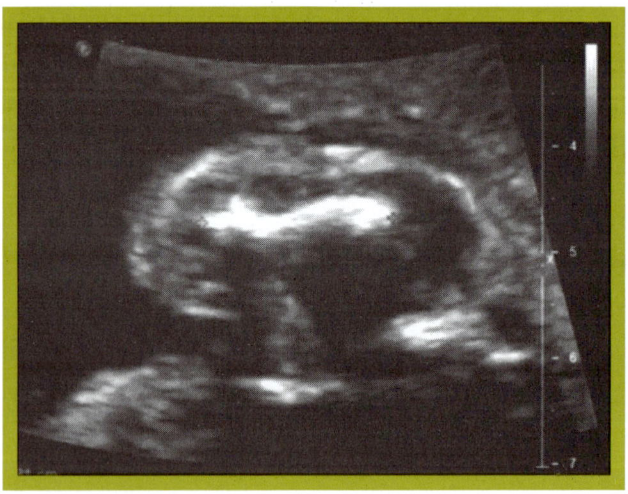

Figure 12.1: Femur in lethal skeletal dysplasia; the femur is short and irregular, showing evidence of intrauterine fractures.

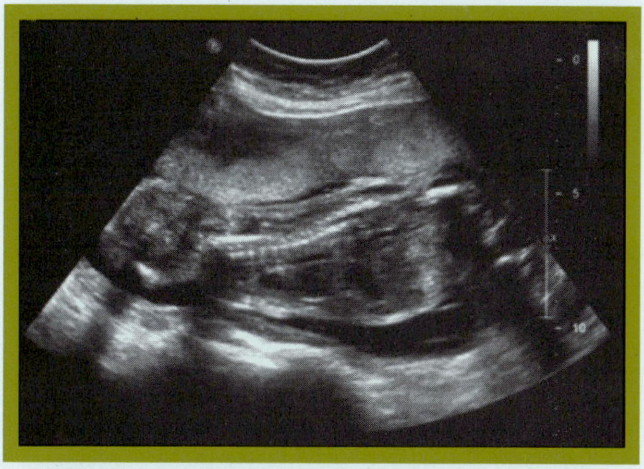

Figure 12.2: Sagittal section of the fetus with lethal skeletal dysplasia; note the significant narrowing of the chest when compared to the abdomen.

with fetal swallowing. Common lethal skeletal dysplasias are thanatophoric dysplasia, osteogenesis imperfecta (type 2), achondrogenesis, hypophosphatasia and homozygous achondroplasia. Each of these conditions may have subtypes. Preterm birth resulting from polyhydramnios is common. Pregnancy termination is reasonable in cases with prenatal diagnosis of lethal skeletal dysplasia. Skeletal shortening is evident from early pregnancy. There is a known association between increased nuchal translucency and lethal skeletal dysplasias (Figs 12.1 and 12.2).

Non-lethal skeletal dysplasias: This is a group of a large number of varieties of skeletal dysplasias. A detailed discussion of each of these is outside the scope of this book, however. Excellent resources such as Online Mendelian Inheritance in Man (OMIM) are available on the internet.

Achondroplasia

This is the most frequent form of short-limb dwarfism. It occurs in 1 in 15,000 to 1 in 40,000 live births. Affected individuals exhibit short stature caused by rhizomelic shortening of the limbs, characteristic facies with frontal bossing and mid-face hypoplasia, exaggerated lumbar lordosis, limitation of elbow extension, genu varum and trident hand.

Achondroplasia is an autosomal dominant disorder; the majority of cases are sporadic, the result of a de novo mutation. Achondroplasia is caused by a

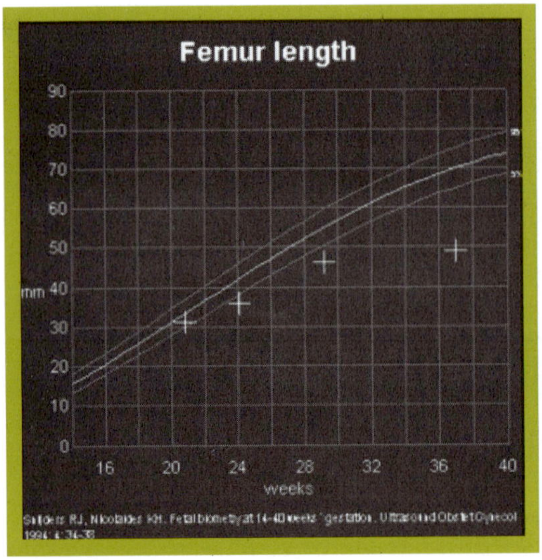

Figure 12.3: Typical growth curve of a fetus with achondroplasia

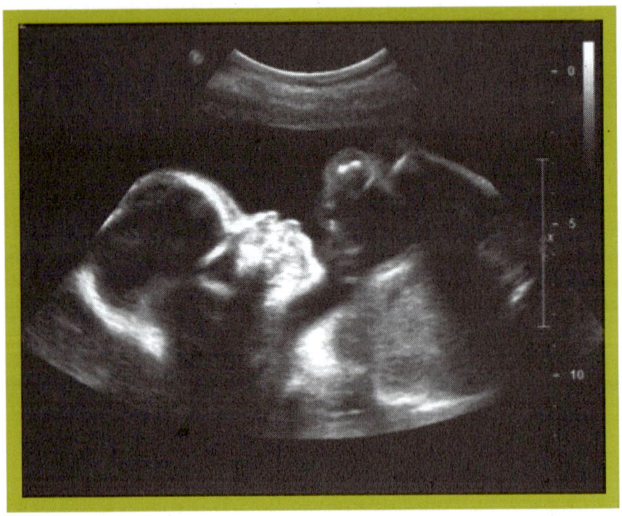

Figure 12.4: Profile of a fetus with achondroplasia; notice the prominent forehead.

mutation in the gene encoding Fibroblast Growth Factor Receptor 3 (FGFR3). Prenatal diagnosis on CVS or amniocentesis is available. Prenatal diagnosis of achondroplasia using ultrasound is not very effective. The FL in most cases of achondroplasia is within the normal range at the time of the 'anomaly scan', which is commonly carried out between 18 and 23 weeks. Two- and three-dimensional ultrasound scans have been used to detect the characteristic facial features and trident hand in affected fetuses. A late diagnosis is not of much use as the gestational age would be beyond the legal limits for pregnancy termination in most countries (Figs 12.3 and 12.4).

Some of the other non-skeletal dysplasias are chondrodysplasia punctata, femur-fibula-ulna (FFU) complex and diastrophic dysplasia.

Approach to a Case of Suspected Skeletal Dysplasia

Statistically, the birth prevalence of skeletal dysplasia is about 5/10,000 against 5/100 in constitutionally small fetuses. Family history of skeletal dysplasia should be sought. Parental stature should be considered. If there has been a previous successful pregnancy, scan measurements in that pregnancy (with a normal child) are very useful for comparison.

First-trimester NT should be reviewed. The CRL should be used to date the pregnancy. The bone echo-texture should be carefully studied. Evidence of intrauterine fractures should be looked for. All the long bones (femur, humerus, radius, ulna, tibia and fibula) may need to be measured on both sides. Polydactyly should be checked for and excluded. The thorax should be visualised to exclude narrowing. Amniotic fluid volume should be evaluated. If skeletal dysplasia is suspected, consultation with a competent clinical geneticist is invaluable.

Further Reading

- Orioli I, E Castilla and J Barbosa-Neto. 1986. The birth prevalence rates for the skeletal dysplasias. *J Med Genet* 23:328–32.

CHAPTER 13

PRESENCE OF A SOFT MARKER ON AN ANOMALY SCAN

Case: A routine anomaly scan was performed mid-pregnancy. No major abnormalities were observed. However, the sonographer identified an echogenic focus in the fetal heart and was concerned that the risk of Down syndrome may be increased.

A soft marker is an ultrasound finding linked to a chromosomal abnormality (mainly Down syndrome) but which does not constitute a fetal abnormality. Several such soft markers are known, and the list is still being compiled. Some of the common soft markers are listed in Table 13.1.

Implications

Identification of a soft marker increases the risk of Down syndrome in a screening programme. The extent of the increase (LR+ve) is not the same with each marker.

Table 13.1: A list of commonly seen soft markers

Choroid plexus cyst	Increased nuchal thickness
Echogenic focus in the heart	Rocker-bottom feet
Short femur	Clinodactyly
Mild renal pelvic dilatation	Brachycephaly
Echogenic bowel	Short nasal bone
Small for gestational age (SGA)	Two-vessel cord
Sandal gap	

Table 13.2: Presence of a sonographic soft marker and risk of Trisomy 21

Soft Marker	Crude Positive LR	Likelihood Ratio of an Isolated Marker
Nuchal fold	53.05	9.8
Short humerus	22.76	4.1
Short femur	7.94	1.6
Hydronephrosis	6.77	1.0
Echogenic focus	6.41	1.1
Echogenic bowel	21.17	3.0
Major defect	32.96	5.2

The presence of more than one marker also increases the probability of Down syndrome. Bayes' theorem can be used to calculate the risk if a soft marker is identified:

Prior odds (Down syndrome risk due to maternal age) X Likelihood ratio = Posterior odds (post-test risk)

Prior odds can be calculated easily from maternal age. The likelihood ratios of several soft markers are known. It is, therefore, relatively straightforward to calculate the post-test odds of a chromosomal abnormality given the maternal age and the soft marker identified (Table 13.2).

Isolated Soft Markers Versus Multiple Soft Markers

The presence of multiple markers increases the risk of chromosomal abnormalities. The higher the number of soft markers, the higher the risk.

A large series looking at structural defects and the presence of soft markers from a referral fetal medicine unit reported that the risk of chromosomal abnormality increases with increasing number of defects identified. Note that the series clubbed structural defects and soft markers together. Also of note is the fact that this was a highly selected population, which is reflected in the high risk of an underlying chromosomal abnormality (Table 13.3).

The performance of soft markers in the presence of a previous screening is very different from that in an unscreened population. This previous screening

Table 13.3: Increase in risk of chromosomal abnormality based on number of risks identified

Number of Defects*	Chromosomal Abnormality
Any	14%
2 or more	29%
3 or more	48%
4 or more	62%
5 or more	70%

* Defect defined as a structural abnormality or a soft marker

might have been with nuchal translucency, serum biochemistry or a combination of the two. Modern screening techniques such as nuchal translucency or serum quadruple screening have a sensitivity of 75–80%. This means that three out of four chromosomally abnormal fetuses would be detected on the basis of the screening and would be screened out. The value of soft markers in the pre-screened population is limited. Many studies report that the risk of Down syndrome would show little increase in the pre-screened population in the presence of a soft marker.

Impact of Soft Markers on Pregnancy

The impact on pregnancy depends on the type of the soft marker. Some soft markers are benign and have little impact (for example, choroid plexus cysts, sandal gap, echogenic focus in the fetal heart; Fig. 13.1), whereas others (short femur, mild renal pelvic dilatation, hyper-echogenic bowel) have other implications as well, and are covered elsewhere (*Chapter 5, Ecogenic Bowel; Chapter 7, Mild Renal Pelvic Dilatation* and *Chapter 12, Shortening of Long Bones*).

Echogenic bowel: Increased bowel echogenicity is a subjective feature. Classically, if the bowel is as echogenic as a fetal bone, the echogenicity should be considered abnormally increased. It is said to be associated with intra-amniotic bleeding and fetal swallowing of echogenic blood. There is a theoretical risk of placental insufficiency, and growth scans at 28 and 36 weeks may be advisable. Increased bowel echogenicity is also a recognised feature

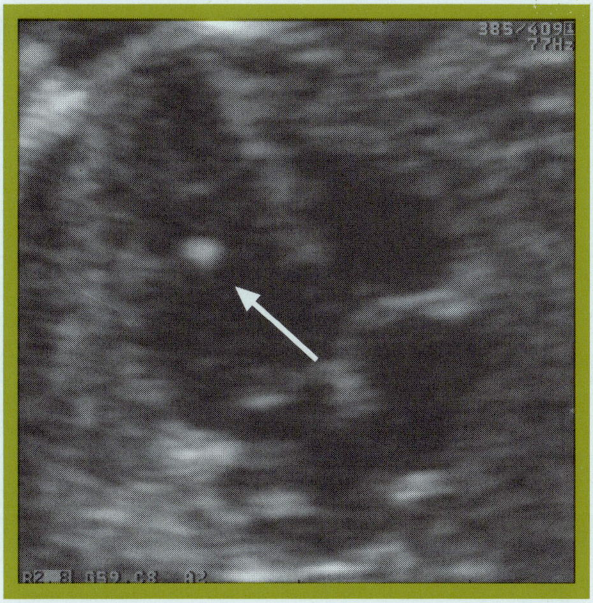

Figure 13.1: Echogenic focus (arrow) in the left ventricle of the fetal heart

of fetal cystic fibrosis. If amniocentesis is carried out, it may be worthwhile screening the amniotic fluid for common mutations (ΔF-508) associated with cystic fibrosis. Echogenic bowel is also a feature of severe fetal growth restriction. However, fetal biometry would almost always be below the reference range by this stage.

Short femur: A short femur is usually defined as FL <5th centile, and as such is expected to be encountered in 5% of the population by definition. This may be due to wrong pregnancy dating, fetal growth restriction, normally grown but constitutionally small fetus or, rarely, fetal skeletal dysplasia. Refer to *Chapter 12, Shortening of Long Bones* for more details.

Mild renal pelvic dilatation: The prevalence of mild renal pelvic dilatation is 2–3% of the population; it is commoner in male fetuses. In the vast majority of cases, renal pelvic dilatation either disappears before or after birth, or remains stable. It may progress in a small minority. Some cases, where it persists after birth, may require post-natal surgery. The probability of post-natal renal surgery is less than 5%. A follow-up scan at about 32 weeks may be advisable (Fig. 13.2).

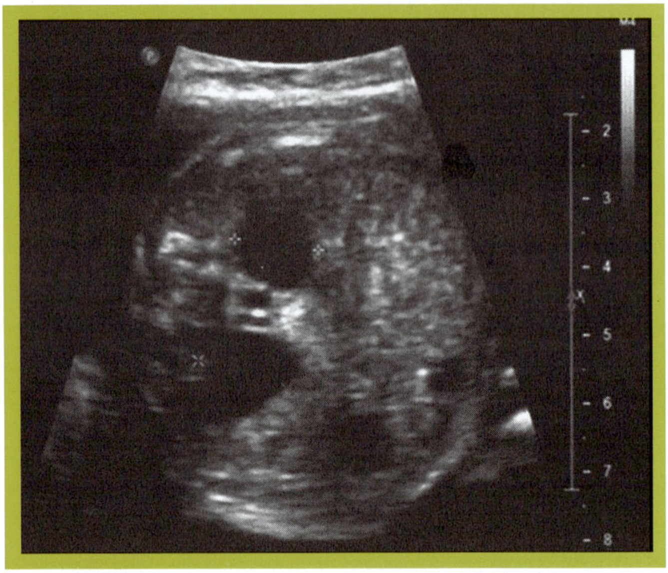

Figure 13.2: Bilateral renal pelvic dilatation seen on the scan

Further Reading

- Cicero S, C Sacchini, G Rembouskos and KH Nicolaides. 2003. Sonographic markers of fetal aneuploidy—A review. *Placenta* 24, S88–S98.
- Nicolaides KH, RJ Snijders, CM Gosden, C Berry and S Campbell. 1992. Ultrasonographically detectable markers of fetal chromosomal abnormalities. *Lancet* 340:704–7.
- Prefumo F, F Presti, E Mavrides, AF Sanusi, JM Bland, S Campbell and JS Carvalho. 2001. Isolated echogenic foci in the fetal heart: Do they increase the risk of trisomy 21 in a population previously screened by nuchal translucency? *Ultrasound Obstet Gynecol* 18:126–30.
- Sairam S, A Al-Habib, S Sasson and B Thilaganathan. 2001. Natural history of fetal hydronephrosis diagnosed on mid-trimester ultrasound. *Ultrasound Obstet Gynecol* 17:191–96.

CHAPTER 14

SUSPECTED FETAL GROWTH RESTRICTION

Case: An ultrasound scan was carried out because the fundal height measurement was less than expected on clinical examination. All the fetal measurements were small on the scan. Good fetal movement was seen. The amniotic fluid volume was somewhat reduced and there was positive end diastolic flow in the umbilical artery.

How Small is Too Small?

The definition of smallness is usually based on statistics. Measurements below the 5th centile are generally considered to be abnormally small. It is best to use the reference range based on a multi-ethnic population, so that the finding is valid despite ethnic differences.

Causes

Dating problems

All fetal measurements are based on the length of gestation, and pregnancy dating is vital. Pregnancies are best dated on crown–rump length (CRL) obtained at 10–14 weeks. It is a national recommendation in many countries to date the pregnancy on CRL even if the menstrual dates are reliably known. (The only exception to this rule is in cases of IVF pregnancies, which are dated on the date of fertilisation). If information about an early pregnancy scan is that known, the pregnancy can be dated on the head circumference or transverse cerebellar diameter (TCD). The dating on fetal biometry is valid till 24 weeks. In general, earlier dating is more reliable. A pregnancy cannot be reliably dated after 24 weeks. In such cases it is impossible to make a diagnosis at the first visit. A follow-up scan and interval growth may be useful.

Placental insufficiency

It is often possible to identify the setting of placental insufficiency. It is more common in the first pregnancy, if the pregnancy is with a new partner, or the previous pregnancy was more than 5 years earlier. Otherwise, there may be a previous history of placental insufficiency or a medical condition that makes placental insufficiency more likely. A typical example is pre-pregnancy hypertension. Uterine arterial Doppler screen is important in such cases. Early onset fetal growth restriction is unusual without an abnormal uterine artery Doppler screen (refer to *Chapter 9, Positive Uterine Artery Doppler Screen*).

Placental insufficiency elicits a typical fetal response. The initial response is the slowing of fetal growth. This slowing, however, is not symmetrical. The fetal abdominal circumference (AC) is more affected than the head circumference (HC). The HC/AC ratio is often abnormal. In very early onset placental insufficiency, all the fetal measurements may be below the 5th centile, but the HC/AC ratio is still abnormal.

The second fetal response is abnormality in fetal Dopplers. There is evidence of fetal blood flow 're-distribution'. Increased resistance in the umbilical artery is seen, whereas the blood flow to the fetal brain increases (low resistance). This results in a rising umbilical artery PI and decreasing middle cerebral artery (MCA) PI. The subsequent response is abnormality in fetal venous Dopplers. This results from fetal decompensation, and is a late change and pre-terminal response. After 34–36 weeks of pregnancy, normal umbilical artery Doppler findings are not reassuring, as fetal compromise may still occur. Middle cerebral artery flow should be evaluated to check for evidence of 're-distribution'.

A typical report of Doppler findings in a growth restricted fetus at 29 weeks is shown below:

Doppler

Umbilical Artery	**PI 3.01** **End diastolic flow: reverse flow**
Middle Cerebral Artery	**PI 1.63** **End diastolic flow: positive**
Ductus Venosus	**PIV 0.880**

Diagnosis

SGA: Likely uteroplacental insufficiency.

The importance of amniotic fluid volume in the diagnosis of placental insufficiency is limited. Amniotic fluid index (AFI) is a semi-quantitative technique of measuring the amniotic fluid. However, it correlates poorly with actual amniotic fluid volume. Prior to the availability of fetal Dopplers, the amniotic fluid volume was of some use. With the availability of fetal Dopplers, use of AFI became superfluous.

Normally grown but small fetus

The diagnosis of a normally grown constitutionally small fetus is one of exclusion. There is no test to establish this diagnosis. The ultrasound features of the initial stage of placental insufficiency and that of a constitutionally small fetus are very similar. Abnormal fetal Dopplers are indicative of placental insufficiency but normal fetal Dopplers do not exclude it. It is only through regular follow-up scans that one can make a reasonably certain diagnosis of a constitutionally small fetus.

Maternal constitution is often indicative of the diagnosis. The fetal size can be 'customised' using maternal demographic parameters and may no longer be below the 5th centile. This requires the use of a specially designed free software (www.gestation.net). The diagnosis of a constitutionally small fetus can never be confirmed. It is desirable to arrange elective delivery closer to the due date and not allow the pregnancy to proceed beyond 41 weeks. In the subgroup of fetuses with birth weight below the 3rd centile and delivered beyond 41 weeks, there is a 38-fold increase in the risk of cerebral palsy.

Intrinsic fetal problems

Intrinsic fetal problems are much less commonly observed. Down syndrome is the commonest chromosomal abnormality but is not associated with abnormal growth. Severe early-onset fetal growth restriction is a feature of fetal triploidy. Trisomy 18 or 13 may also be associated with fetal growth restriction. Many other markers of chromosomal abnormality may be observed in the fetus and include heart defects, other abnormalities such as exomphalos or facial clefting, polydactyly, abnormal skull shape or talipes. Some genetic syndromes such as Smith–Lemli–Opitz or Russell–Silver are also known to be associated with fetal growth restriction. The typical features are significant growth restriction (biometry <3rd centile) with no risk factors and normal uterine artery and fetal Dopplers.

Congenital viral infections are a known but rare association. Congenital rubella syndrome and congenital CMV or toxoplasmosis infection lead to significant growth restriction. A history of exposure to the infection may be present. Other features include microcephaly, ventriculomegaly and echogenicities in the periventricular area and fetal liver. The outlook is extremely guarded. Maternal cocaine abuse can also lead to fetal growth restriction. The drug can cause intense vasospasm and lead to both congenital abnormalities and intrauterine demise. Maternal alcohol abuse is linked with fetal growth restriction, but there is no definitive test available for confirming the diagnosis.

Suspected fetal growth restriction: When to deliver

The time of delivery depends on the exact cause of the smallness. Elective early delivery is likely to be beneficial only in cases of smallness due to placental insufficiency.

In general, absence of end diastolic flow in the umbilical artery is an indication for delivery after 34 weeks. Reversed end diastolic flow in the umbilical artery should prompt delivery at 32 weeks and after. Before 32 weeks, the risks from prematurity are substantial, and even a few days gained in utero are likely to significantly improve prematurity risks. The timing of delivery in such cases should be very carefully determined. It is based on CTG changes or changes in the flow velocity waveforms in the fetal ductus venosus.

Delivery before 28 weeks may not be associated with intact survival, even with administration of maternal steroids. As a rule, an estimated fetal weight of 500 g and maturity of 28 weeks is required for delivery.

Beyond 34 weeks, and till 37 weeks, delivery would be indicated for increased resistance in the umbilical artery, with reduction of resistance in the fetal middle cerebral artery (fetal brain sparing or blood flow redistribution). Beyond 37 weeks, significant fetal compromise is possible even without frankly abnormal umbilical artery Doppler.

Further Reading

- Badawi N, JJ Kurinczuk, JM Keogh, LM Alessandri, F O'Sullivan, PR Burton, PJ Pemberton and FJ Stanley. 1998. Antepartum risk factors for newborn encephalopathy: The Western Australian case-control study. *BMJ* 317:1549–53.
- Hershkovitz R, JC Kingdom, M Geary and CH Rodeck. 2000. Fetal cerebral blood flow redistribution in late gestation: Identification of compromise in small fetuses with normal umbilical artery Doppler. *Ultrasound Obstet Gynecol* 15:209–12.
- Severi FM, C Bocchi, A Visentin, P Falco, L Cobellis, P Florio, S Zagonari and G Pilu. 2002. Uterine and fetal cerebral Doppler predict the outcome of third-trimester small-for-gestational age fetuses with normal umbilical artery Doppler. *Ultrasound Obstet Gynecol* 19:225–28.

CHAPTER 15

TWIN-TO-TWIN TRANSFUSION SYNDROME

Case: A 28-year-old woman was known to be carrying twins. She was referred for a scan at 22 weeks in view of a sudden increase in the size of the bump. The uterus was tense, and she could not be comfortable in any position. The ultrasound scan showed a twin pregnancy with both heartbeats. However, the inter-twin membrane could not be visualised. The question of a monoamniotic pregnancy was raised. There was marked polyhydramnios.

Twin-to-twin transfusion syndrome (TTTS) is a complication seen in approximately 15% of monochorionic twin pregnancies. There has been a lot of progress in the understanding of the pathophysiology of this condition. This complication develops only in monochorionic twin pregnancies. Therefore, accurate assignment of chorionicity in early pregnancy (refer to *Chapter 2, Twin Gestation and Invasive Testing*) is vital.

TTTS can be classified according to a staging system first described by Quintero et al.

Stage I: Discrepancy in liquor volume only. Oligohydramnios (maximum vertical pocket <2 cm) in the donor, and polyhydramnios (maximum vertical pocket >8 cm) in the recipient (Fig. 15.1). Fetal bladder in the donor is still demonstrable in Stage 1.

Stage II: Absent bladder in the donor, big bladder in the recipient. Fetal Dopplers are still not critical (Fig. 15.2).

Stage III: Critically abnormal arterial Dopplers. Absent-to-reversed end diastolic flow in the umbilical artery of the donor twin; reversed

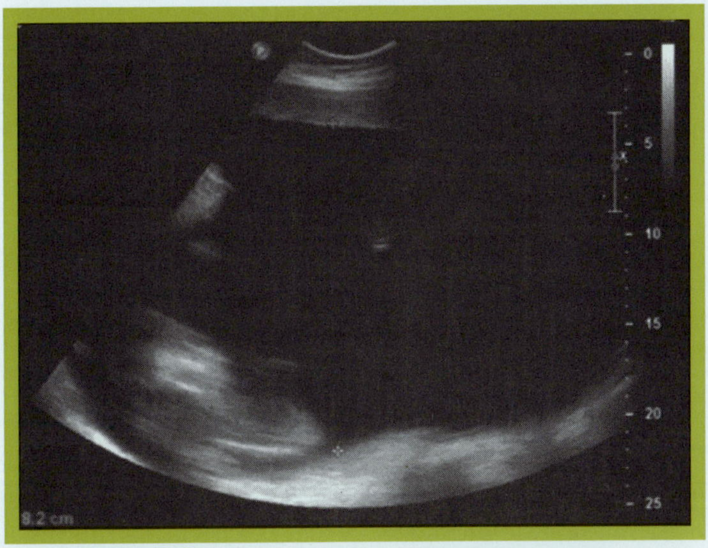

Figure 15.1: Gross polyhydramnios in a case of TTTS

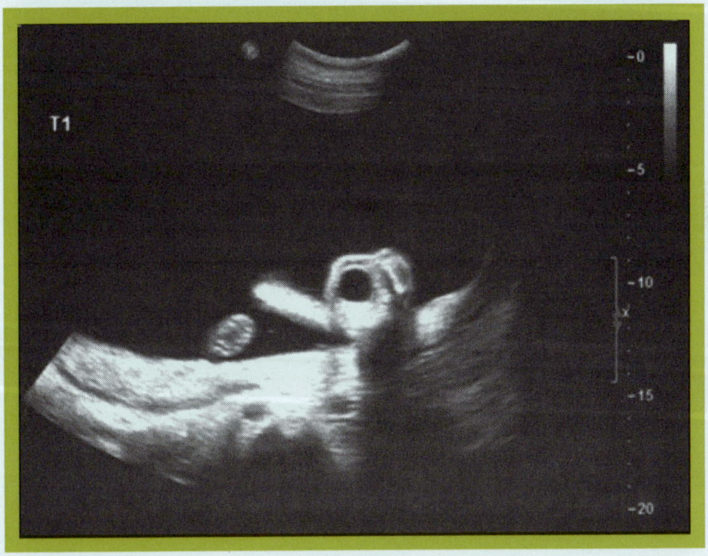

Figure 15.2: Donor fetus demonstrating a big urinary bladder in a case of TTTS; note the presence of excessive amniotic fluid.

'a' wave in the ductus venosus or pulsatile flow in the umbilical vein of the recipient twin (Fig. 15.3).

Stage IV: Presence of hydrops fetalis in the recipient twin (Fig. 15.4).

Stage V: Intrauterine death of one or both twins.

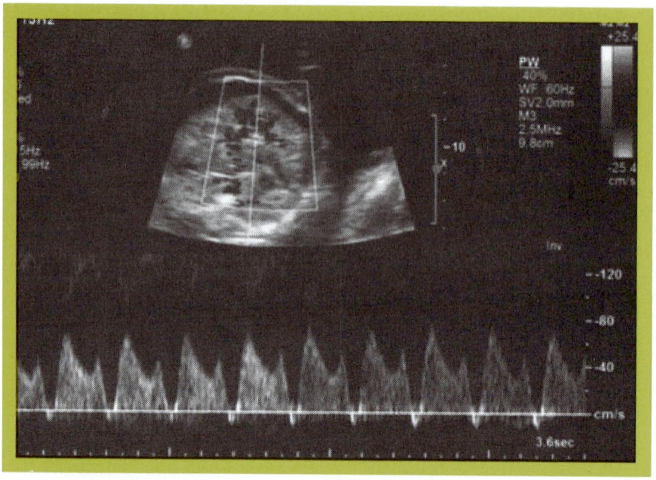

Figure 15.3: Abnormal PI (pulsatility index) in the ductus venosus of the recipient in TTTS

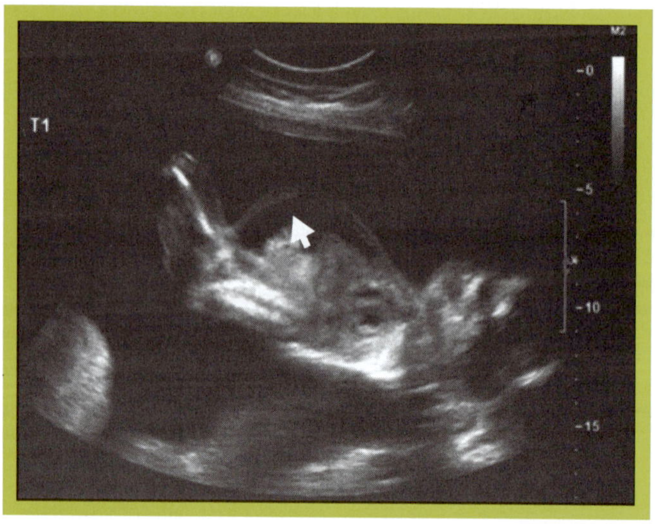

Figure 15.4: Recipient fetus showing presence of hydrops (arrow) in TTTS

Treatment

Observation: Simple observation in a case of progressive TTTS is not advisable. There is a serious risk of spontaneous preterm delivery/late miscarriage in untreated cases. The risk of intrauterine death of one of the monochorionic twins is also present. This is associated with a 25% risk of death of the co-twin and another 25% risk of neurological handicap in the survivor. This is thought to result from significant and sudden fetal anemia in the survivor. Natural history of TTTS is not well-established. There is over-representation of mild cases (Quintero Stage 1), which do not progress and which are associated with a reasonably good outcome. The risk of fetal loss (miscarriage or intrauterine death) in more advanced stages (Quintero Stages 2 and 3) is high, and ranges from 50% to 100%.

Observation is the strategy of choice in cases where the TTTS is mild (Quintero Stage I or II) and not progressive.

Serial amniodrainage: This technique has the advantage of being widely available, simple to perform and capable of reducing the risk of spontaneous preterm labour. It may also improve placental perfusion by relieving pressure on the vessels on the chorionic plate. Using this technique, survival rates of 18–83% (depending on the Quintero stage) have been reported. However, neurological morbidity was reported in 5–58% of survivors. In a large randomised controlled trial of amniodrainage versus laser photocoagulation, there was significant advantage in both survival and intact survival for the latter.

Laser photocoagulation: This procedure involves the use of fetoscopic laser to coagulate the chorionic plate vessels interconnecting the twins. This procedure requires skill and is not very widely available. However, current evidence indicates that this is the procedure of choice for progressive TTTS of Quintero Stages II or higher.

Delivery: This is not a very practical option. Progressive TTTS typically develops after 16 weeks, till 22–24 weeks. Delivery at this stage is associated with severe prematurity.

Cord occlusion of one of the twins: Selective feticide in a monochorionic pregnancy can be achieved by bipolar coagulation of the cord of one of the fetuses. This technique is useful in cases of TTTS where one of the twins shows a structural defect, either as a cause or the effect of TTTS. This requires specially made thin bipolar forceps, which are used under ultrasound guidance. This limits the use of this technique. The technique may also be used in cases where fetoscopic laser is technically difficult as in cases with an anterior placenta. In a series of 46 procedures performed for a variety of indications, preterm rupture of membranes within 4 weeks (10%) and fetal anemia requiring intrauterine transfusion in the survivor (6%) were the main complications.

Septostomy: Septostomy is a relatively new technique in which the inter-twin septum is divided on purpose to achieve equality of amniotic fluid volume. It is difficult to understand how equalising amniotic fluid volume would lead to correction of the inter-twin blood flow. This technique is not widely studied, and there is lack of good quality evidence to support it. Theoretically, this procedure creates an iatrogenic monoamnionic twin pregnancy, which can lead to cord entanglement.

Differential Diagnosis

Chronic progressive TTTS should be differentiated from two other similar conditions: selective fetal growth restriction in a monochorionic twin pair and acute inter-twin transfusion episode.

Selective fetal growth restriction can occur in a monochorionic twin pregnancy. The growth restricted fetus is significantly smaller than its co-twin. The amniotic fluid volume around this fetus is low. However, the normally grown fetus does not show polyhydramnios, and the smaller fetus is rarely 'stuck'. The fetal Dopplers are usually normal in the normally grown twin, but are abnormal in the growth-restricted twin.

Acute inter-twin transfusion episode is a one-off event of twin-twin transfusion that can occur in a monochorionic twin pregnancy. It is unpredictable and not preventable. If a very large volume has been transfused, intrauterine fetal death can result. Table 15.1 illustrates the differentiating features.

The ideal treatment for these conditions is unknown. An acute inter-twin transfusion episode is non-progressive. However, it is impossible to predict whether or when another episode will take place. The next episode may be more severe and lead to in utero death (IUD) of one or more fetuses. Therefore, if the gestational age is beyond 34 weeks, delivery may be advisable. If the gestational age is below 24 weeks, fetoscopic laser should be strongly considered.

The treatment of selective IUGR is also difficult. If the growth restriction is so severe as to cause an in utero death, handicap or death of the co-twin is a

Table 15.1: Differences in the features of the differential diagnoses of TTTS

	Feature	Chronic TTTS	Acute Inter-twin Transfusion Episode	Selective Growth Restriction
Smaller twin	Biometry	Biometry below average, but usually within normal range	Biometry below average, but usually within normal range	Biometry usually below the normal range
	Amniotic fluid	Complete anhydramnios (stuck twin)	May have anhydramnios	Reduced, but unusual to have anhydramnios
	Urinary bladder	Absent	Usually present	Present
	Umbilical artery PI	High	May be normal	Very high
Larger twin	Amniotic fluid	Polyhydramnios	Polyhydramnios	Normal
	Urinary bladder	Big	Normal or big	Normal
	Ductus venosus PI	Usually raised	May be normal	Normal
Progression		Yes	No	Yes (in the smaller fetus)

distinct possibility. Again, elective delivery is the preferred option if maturity is reasonable. Fetoscopic laser or bipolar cord occlusion of the smaller twin may be considered if there is severe early-onset growth restriction in one of the monochorionic twin pairs.

Further Reading

- Fox C, M Kilby and K Khan. 2005. Contemporary treatments for twin–twin transfusion syndrome. *Obstet Gynecol* 105:1469–77.
- Quintero RA, WJ Morales, MH Allen, PW Bornick, PK Johnson and M Kruger. 1999. Staging of twin-twin transfusion syndrome. *J Perinatol* 19:550–55.

Further Reading

- Robyr R, M Yamamoto and Y Ville. 2005. Selective feticide in complicated monochorionic twin pregnancies using ultrasound-guided bipolar cord coagulation. *Br J Obstet Gynaecol* 112:1344–48.
- Senat MV, J Deprest, M Boulvain, A Paupe, N Winer and Y Ville. 2004. Endoscopic laser surgery versus serial amnioreduction for severe twin-to-twin transfusion syndrome. *N Engl J Med* 351:136–44.
- van Gemert M, A Umura, J Tijssen and M Ross. 2001. Twin-twin transfusion syndrome: Etiology, severity and rational management. *Curr Opin Obstet Gynecol* 13:193–206.

CHAPTER 16

MONOCHORIONIC TWIN PREGNANCY

Case: A 27-year-old woman underwent a dating scan at 13 weeks of pregnancy. Two fetuses were identified. A single posterior placenta was seen. The sonographer was unsure if the twins were identical.

It is now widely recognised that the risk in twin pregnancy is related to the chorionicity rather than zygocity. Zygocity is not always easy to detect without the use of molecular biology techniques. All monochorionic pregnancies are monozygotic. However, dichorionic pregnancies may or may not be dizygotic, some of these being monozygotic. All dizygotic pregnancies are dichorionic, but the converse is not true.

The key feature of a monochorionic twin pregnancy is the sharing of the placenta. Monochorionic twin pregnancies, by definition, have a functionally single placenta, and share the placental vasculature. Vascular anastomoses in the placenta are universal. Dichorionic twins have functionally distinct placentas, although these placentas may be fused and appear as a single placenta. Vascular anastomoses are not seen. The increase in fetal risk, unique complications of monochorionicity and management principles are related to the chorionicity.

Increase in Perinatal Mortality

The increase in fetal loss in monochorionic pregnancies is early rather than late. In a large study, there was a higher rate of fetal loss before 24 weeks of gestation in monochorionic than in dichorionic pregnancies (12.2% versus 1.8%).

The perinatal mortality (2.8% versus 1.6%) and prevalence of delivery before 32 weeks (9.2% versus 5.5%) were also increased, although not as dramatically.

Unique Complications of Monochorionicity

- Twin-to-twin transfusion syndrome (TTTS); refer to *Chapter 15* for a detailed account.
- The etiopathology of selective fetal growth restriction and TTTS are very similar. Being monozygotic, the genetic potential for both embryos should be the same. Therefore, any discordance in the weights of the monochorionic twin pair would be abnormal and selective fetal growth restriction difficult to define. Studies focussing on this problem have identified three groups:
  a) birth weight <10th centile or AC <5th centile of one of the twins
  b) birth weight discordance (difference in weight>15% of the weight of the bigger twin)
  c) abdominal circumference <5th centile in combination with absent or reversed end diastolic (ARED) flow in the umbilical artery of one of the twins (Fig. 16.1).
- Studies have reported that the prevalence of selective growth restriction in mono and dichorionic pregnancies is similar. The prevalence of severe birth weight discordance (difference in weight >25% of the larger twin weight)

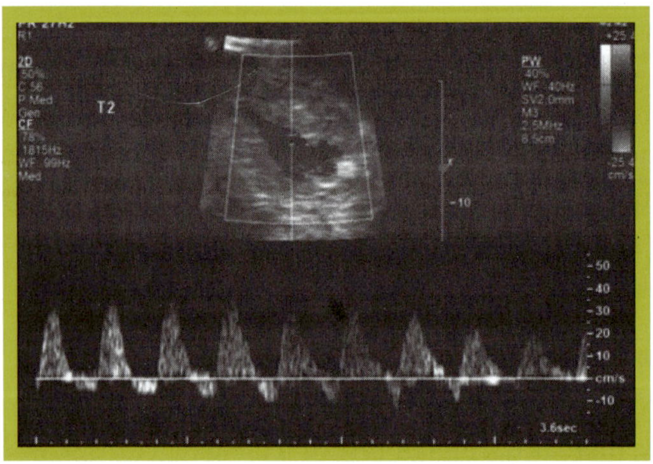

Figure 16.1: Intermittent absent reversed end diastolic flow in the umbilical artery of the smaller twin

was similar in both mono and dichorionic twins. However, the outcome was much worse in monochorionic twins. A study on selective IUGR in monochorionic twins with the smaller twin exhibiting intermittent absent/ reversed end diastolic blood flow reported that there was a 20% risk of intrauterine death. There also was a 20% risk of brain damage, mostly in the non–growth restricted baby.

- Another study reported that amniotic fluid discordance in monochorionic diamniotic twin pregnancies in combination with IUGR and umbilical artery ARED flow in one fetus represents an extremely high-risk constellation for adverse pregnancy outcome. The overall survival in this group was only 60% (92% in the control group). Bipolar cord coagulation of the growth-restricted twin and fetoscopic laser separation of the placenta are two treatment options. The ideal treatment option for this group is unknown at present.
- In dichorionic twin pregnancies, in utero demise of one of the twins has little impact on the survival of its co-twin. Indeed, if one of the dichorionic twins shows signs of severe early-onset fetal growth restriction and there is a significant risk of spontaneous intrauterine death, the standard advice is to defer intervention till at least 32 weeks. Elective delivery after 32 weeks (with prior maternal steroid administration) is unlikely to pose significant risks to the normally grown twin. In dichorionic twins, however, single intrauterine death poses a serious risk of death or handicap to the surviving co-twin due to the presence of vascular anastomoses. In monochorionic twin gestations complicated by TTTS and fetal death of one twin, approximately half of the surviving twins will experience mortality or serious morbidity. In a study of 20 monochorionic twins with the intrauterine death of one, 10/20 survivors were anemic when investigated within 24 hours of the event. It has now emerged that sudden blood loss from the surviving twin is likely to be at least partially responsible for the poor outlook of the survivor. Rescue transfusions to the surviving twin have been reported, but the utility of this approach is unproven.
- Conjoint twinning is a very rare complication of monochorionic twins. The outlook is related to the presence of shared organs and is generally guarded. Complex surgical procedures may need to be done to separate the

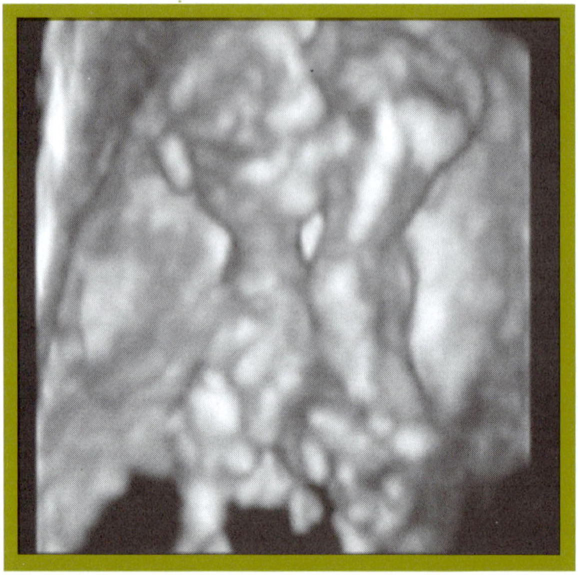

Figure 16.2: A 3D image of conjoint twins at 13 weeks

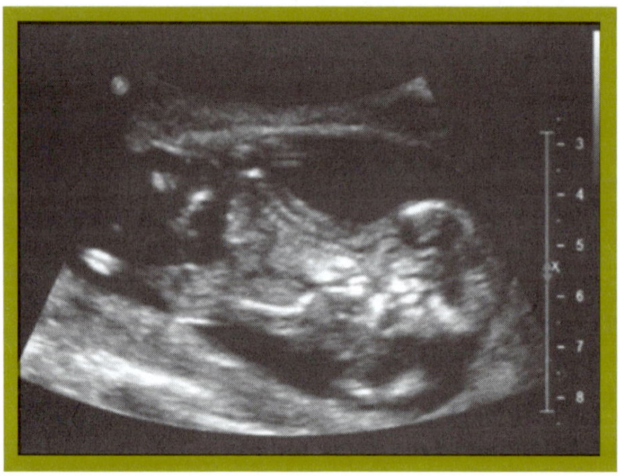

Figure 16.3: A greyscale image of conjoint twins. Note the close approximation of the twins. The twins fail to move away from each other on prolonged scanning, even with fetal movement.

twins after birth. Delivery itself can be very complex, and an elective (often classical) cesarean section may be necessary. Figures 16.2 and 16.3 show a case of conjoint twins identified at 13 weeks of pregnancy.

- Twin-reversed arterial perfusion (TRAP) is a unique complication of monochorionicity and occurs in approximately 1% of monochorionic twins. In early pregnancy, the presence of arterioarterial and venovenous anastomosis between both cord insertions in monochorionic twins may lead to a reversal of perfusion through the umbilical artery of one twin, if one pulse wave predominates over the other early in gestation. In the reversely perfused twin, there is no cardiac development at all or only a rudimentary heart tube can be detected. The development of the upper part of the body is also severely impaired and most of the acardiac fetuses show acrania and severe hydrops. The natural history of the TRAP sequence is that of a guarded outlook. TRAP is associated with a high risk of heart failure and intrauterine demise or preterm delivery of the pump twin. In the largest series (49 acardiac twin pregnancies without intrauterine surgery), mortality for the pump twin was 51% and delivery occurred in only 24% after 36 weeks' gestation. Several techniques have been described for treatment, and the choice of treatment and timing are uncertain. Successful expectant management of selected cases has been described. Invasive treatment should be restricted to pregnancies that would potentially benefit from prenatal intervention. It has been suggested that in utero invasive treatment should be considered only in cases in which poor prognostic factors are detected, including the development of polyhydramnios, ultrasound markers of cardiac insufficiency (that is, tricuspid regurgitation, pulsatile umbilical vein and abnormal ductus venosus waveforms in the pump twin's circulation),

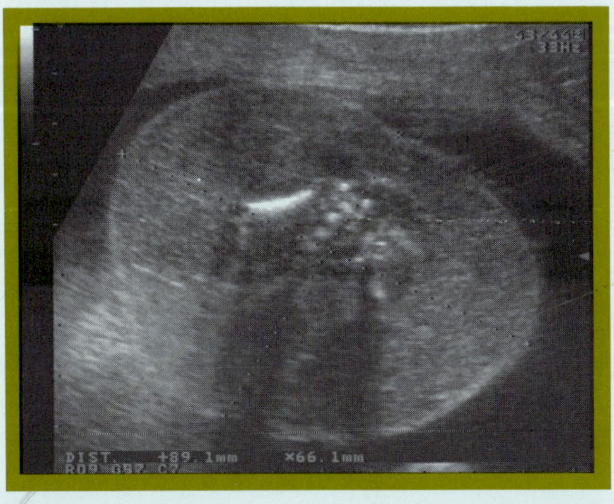

Figure 16.4: A TRAP twin; note the presence of massive edema.

large acardiac twin and rapid growth of, or evidence of, substantial blood flow perfusion through the umbilical vessel supplying the parasitic mass. Fetoscopic techniques (cord ligation, laser) carry a higher risk of preterm birth than the minimally invasive ones (interstitial laser, injection of sclerosing liquids). Figure 16.4 shows a TRAP twin.

- It has been shown that multiple inter-twin vascular communications protect against the development of TTTS. However, this may pose a problem to the twins at delivery. After the delivery of the first twin, the second twin may 'bleed' in the common placenta and be born with significant anemia. The volume loss is likely to be proportional to the number and calibre of inter-twin communications and the inter-twin delivery time interval. A policy of elective cesarean delivery for all monochorionic twins is defended on this ground. If vaginal delivery is attempted, careful monitoring of the second twin should be carried out after delivery of the first.

Further Reading

- Bhide A, F Prefumo, S Sairam, F Cobian-Sanchez and B Thilaganathan. 2006. Effect of inter-twin delivery interval on neonatal haemoglobin concentration. *J Obstet Gynaecol* 26:759–62.
- Gratacos E, E Carreras, J Becker, L Lewi, G Enriquez, J Perapoch, T Higueras, L Cabero and J Deprest. 2004. Prevalence of neurological damage in monochorionic twins with selective intrauterine growth restriction and intermittent absent or reversed end-diastolic umbilical artery flow. *Ultrasound Obstet Gynecol* 24:159–63.
- Moore TR, S Gale and K Benirschke. 1990. Perinatal outcome of forty nine pregnancies complicated by acardiac twinning. *Am J Obstet Gynecol* 163:907–12.
- Sebire NJ, RJ Snijders, K Hughes, W Sepulveda and KH Nicolaides. 1997. The hidden mortality of monochorionic twin pregnancies. *Br J Obstet Gynaecol* 104:1203–7.
- Sepulveda W and N Sebire. 2004. Acardiac twin: Too many invasive treatment options—the problem and not the solution. *Ultrasound Obstet Gynecol* 24: 387–89.

CHAPTER 17

RED CELL ALLOIMMUNISATION

Case: An ultrasound scan was performed because the fundal height was greater than expected. A single live fetus was seen with no major structural abnormalities. There was evidence of increase in amniotic fluid volume. The ultrasound features raised suspicions of fetal anemia. The clinical features were consistent with red cell alloimmunisation. However, the mother was rhesus-positive.

Erythroblastosis fetalis is a disease in which the red cells of the fetus and the newborn are destroyed by maternal alloantibodies that cross the placenta. With the widespread use of anti-D prophylaxis, anti-D alloimmunisation is less common, and in a significant proportion of cases, the cause is other atypical antigens, notably Kell, c and E. Maternal alloimmunisation is usually detected by routine antenatal screening for the presence of atypical antibodies. Atypical antibodies should be looked for in all women, and not only those who are rhesus-negative. In the United Kingdom, this is a routine practice at booking and again at 28 weeks of pregnancy. As yet, this has not been made routine for rhesus-positive women in some other countries. It is worthwhile requesting this test if the mother has a history of prolonged/ exaggerated jaundice in an earlier baby or of blood transfusions at birth. The antibodies may also develop if the mother has been transfused with blood or blood products in the past.

The management of alloimmunised patients is based on the appropriate use of maternal serum antibody levels, fetal assessment by ultrasound scan and fetal blood sampling.

Maternal Serum Antibody Levels

In cases of sensitisation against the D antigen in the first affected pregnancy, the antibody levels correlate well with the likelihood of fetal anemia. Significant fetal anemia is uncommon with anti-D levels below 15 IU/ml. Several laboratories have developed a 'critical titre', a titre below which no case of death due to erythroblastosis fetalis was encountered within one week of that antibody titre. The antibody levels are tested from 16 weeks till 28 weeks at 4-weekly intervals, and every two weeks thereafter. A significant rise in the titre (a more than fourfold rise in titre or anti-D levels of 15 IU/ml or more) is suggestive of fetal anemia. In subsequent pregnancies, history plays an important role. In general, the antibody level at which fetal anemia was detected in the previous pregnancy is likely to lead to fetal anemia in the subsequent pregnancy as well. If the anti-D titre remains below 15 IU/ml and there are no ultrasound features of fetal anemia at all times up to 36 weeks, elective delivery should be arranged after 37 weeks. If the titre shows a significant rise, or if ultrasound features raise suspicions of fetal anemia, elective delivery is advisable after 34 weeks after maternal steroid administration rather than fetal blood sampling and intrauterine transfusion, due to the risks of the invasive procedures.

It is possible to predict the rhesus group of the fetus by analysing the free fetal DNA in maternal circulation. This is particularly important if the father is heterozygous for the D antigen (Dd), because there is a 1:2 chance that the fetus will be rhesus-negative and, therefore, unaffected regardless of the antibody levels.

Fetal Assessment by Ultrasound

Ultrasound scans can detect ascites, pericardial and pleural effusions, hepatomegaly, skin edema and placental enlargement. Excessive fluid collection at any two sites is termed hydrops fetalis. Typically, hydrops occurs when the hemoglobin deficit exceeds 6 gm%. These ultrasound features are late signs signifying severe fetal anemia (Fig. 17.1). The survival of fetuses with established hydrops is significantly worse than those without, even with treatment by intrauterine transfusion. There is some evidence to suggest that fetuses with severe anemia may have an inferior neurological outcome than those without.

Non-invasive diagnosis of fetal anemia using Doppler ultrasound has radically altered the management of fetal anemia due to alloimmunisation. This is based on the principle that fetal anemia reduces the viscosity of fetal blood,

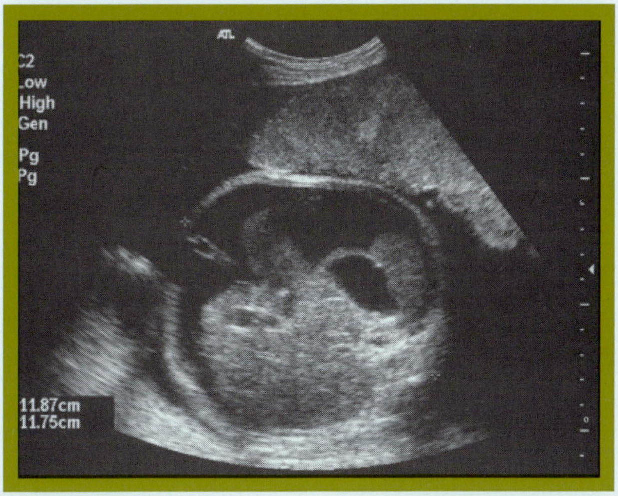

Figure 17.1: Transverse section through fetal abdomen; note the collection of fluid in the fetal abdomen as an anechoic space.

allowing it to move fast. The peak systolic velocity of fetal blood correlates well with the hematocrit. Accurate measurement of peak systolic velocity is the key. Technically, measurement of peak systolic velocity in the middle cerebral artery (MCA-PSV) is associated with the least error, and is clinically useful (Fig. 17.2).

The MCA-PSV changes with advancing gestation. Reference ranges for MCA-PSV have been published. Mari, using a cut-off of 0.6 multiples of median (MOM) above the mean, reported a sensitivity of 100% for the detection of fetal

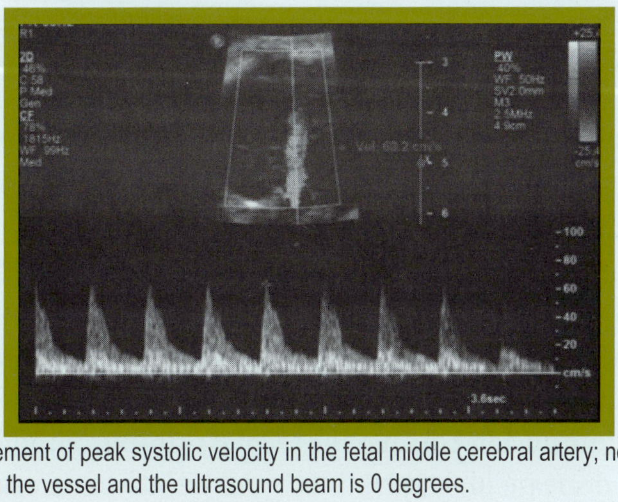

Figure 17.2: Measurement of peak systolic velocity in the fetal middle cerebral artery; note that the angle between the vessel and the ultrasound beam is 0 degrees.

anemia. The positive predictive value in his study was 12%. This means that only 1 in 8 fetuses with suspected anemia sampled were in fact anemic. A higher cut-off of MCA-PSV would probably increase the positive predictive value at the expense of missing some cases of mild-to-moderate fetal anemia. In the author's centre, a cut-off of the 95th centile was used for MCA-PSV.

Fetal Blood Sampling

When there is a risk of fetal anemia as demonstrated by an increase in the antibody titre, a rise in the MCA-PSV above the chosen cut-off or if the mother is complaining of fetal movement reduction, intervention is mandated. If elective preterm delivery is not an acceptable option (gestational age below 34 weeks), fetal blood sampling should be scheduled under ultrasound guidance. The use of fetal blood sampling, first described by Daffos et al, allows direct estimation of fetal hematocrit, blood group and direct Coomb's test. Arrangements for simultaneous intrauterine transfusion must be made should fetal anemia be confirmed. This involves sending a maternal blood sample to the blood bank prior to the scheduled procedure for cross-matched, irradiated packed red blood cells. Irradiation destroys the white blood cells so as to avoid the possibility of a graft versus host reaction. A needle is guided in the placental insertion of the umbilical vein under real-time ultrasound control, and a blood sample is collected for measurement of hemoglobin. This is compared to the gestational age–adjusted reference range previously published, in order to quantify the deficit. An appropriate volume of compatible packed red cells is transfused in the umbilical vein. The volume depends on the hematocrit of the fetus and that of the packed cells (typically Hb >24 g/dl), as well as the gestational age.

Maternal antibody titre invariably rises as a result of the needling, and there is no purpose in serial titre measurements. The fetus remains at risk of developing anemia and is likely to require a second transfusion after 10–14 days. This too can be timed on the basis of measurements of fetal MCA-PSV. The MCA-PSV is not useful in predicting severe anemia in fetuses that have already had two previous transfusions. The only significant predictor of fetal anemia in patients who have received two previous transfusions is the estimation of the Hb from the measured post-transfusion Hb after the second transfusion, and the assumption that the rate of decrease in fetal Hb is 0.3 g/dl per day. Every procedure of fetal blood sampling and intrauterine transfusion is associated with a risk of preterm delivery, and prophylactic glucocorticoids are indicated if the procedure is carried out after 24 weeks. In the rare case where significant fetal affliction is suspected prior to 20–22 weeks, fetal intravascular transfusion is technically difficult. Intraperitoneal transfusion can be carried out till such time that safe intravascular transfusion becomes technically possible.

Care at Delivery

Delivery should take place at a centre capable of managing frequent bilirubin estimations, phototherapy and exchange transfusions. Delivery should be planned, if possible, and the neonatologists and experts in transfusion medicine alerted beforehand. Compatible blood, cross-matched against maternal serum, should be kept ready at delivery in the event of a requirement for exchange transfusion at birth. Administration of a large dose of intravenous IgG immunoglobulin can be used to achieve 'immune paralysis' by saturation of the receptors of the fetal reticulo-endothelial system and to delay destruction of fetal red cells, thereby preventing severe jaundice. Cord blood sample should be collected for hematocrit, bilirubin and direct Coomb's test.

Further Reading

- Daffos F, M Capalla-Pavlovsky and F Forrestier. 1983. A new procedure for fetal blood sampling in utero: Preliminary result of fifty-three cases. *Am J Obstet Gynecol* 146:985–87.
- Mari G, A Ardignolo, A Abuhamad, J Pirhonen, D Jones, A Ludomirsky and J Copel. 1995. Diagnosis of fetal anemia using Doppler ultrasound in the pregnancy complicated by maternal blood group immunisation. *Ultrasound Obstet Gynecol* 5:400–405.
- Moise K. 2006. Diagnosing hemolytic disease of the fetus—time to put the needles away? *N Engl J Med* 355:192–94.
- Scheier M, E Hernandes-Andrade, E Fonseca and K Nicolaides. 2006. Prediction of severe fetal anemia in red blood cell alloimmunization after previous intrauterine transfusions. *Am J Obstet Gynecol* 195:1550–56.

CHAPTER 18

HYDROPS FETALIS

Case: An ultrasound scan was performed because the fundal height was greater than expected. A single live fetus was seen. There was ultrasound evidence of fluid collection in the chest and abdomen. No other major structural abnormalities were seen. There was evidence of increase in amniotic fluid volume. The mother was rhesus-positive. .

Technically, excessive fluid collection in two or more body cavities is defined as hydrops fetalis. This may constitute hydrothorax, pericardial effusion, ascites, skin edema, cystic hygroma or a combination thereof. Hydrops fetalis is not a diagnosis, but may result from a variety of underlying problems. These can be grouped as follows:

- Immune fetal anemia—red cell alloimmunisation (refer to *Chapter 17, Red Cell Alloimmunisation*)
- Chromosomal abnormalities
- Fetal infections—parvovirus B19 infection, congenital CMV, toxoplasma/ rubella infection
- Cardiac arrhythmias—atrial flutter/SVT, congenital complete heart block
- Genetic metabolic causes—storage disorders, mitochondrial disorders
- Hematological disorders—alpha thalassemia, rare hemoglobinopathies
- Complication of monochorionic twin pregnancy—twin-to-twin transfusion syndrome, TRAP twin (refer to *Chapter 2, Twin Gestation and Invasive Testing* and *Chapter 15, Twin-to-Twin Transfusion Syndrome*)

Immune fetal anemia: It is unusual for hydrops fetalis caused by red cell alloimmunisation to come to light for the first time as a result of an ultrasound examination. The common practice is to check the blood group and presence of atypical antibodies at the time of antenatal booking. There may be a history of previous babies with jaundice and anemia or intrauterine deaths. An anemic fetus exhibits a reduction in movement, and this may be evident on history. The use of peak systolic velocity in the middle cerebral artery is invaluable in the assessment of suspected fetal anemia, as detailed in *Chapter 17, Red Cell Alloimmunisation*. It is important to note that rhesus positivity does not eliminate red cell alloimmunisation, as a significant proportion of women will have antibodies against non-rhesus antigens.

Chromosomal abnormalities: The risk of chromosomal abnormality can be assessed by the mother's age, previous nuchal translucency measurement and presence of other soft markers or abnormalities. In a series of 51 cases of intrauterine hydrops fetalis identified prior to 24 weeks, chromosomal abnormalities were present in 23 (45%).

Fetal infections: Fetal infections due to toxoplasma, CMV or parvovirus can manifest as hydrops fetalis. The mechanism is not the same though. Fetal parvovirus infection leads to hydrops as a combination of fetal anemia and viral myocarditis (Fig. 18.1). Again, the finding of MCA-PSV above the 95th centile and enlargement of the fetal heart are supportive findings. The infection is usually self-limiting, as the fetus mounts an immune response. However, an intrauterine transfusion may be required to tide over the critical period before an adequate immune response has been achieved. In a recent study of 16 survivors of parvovirus infection treated with intrauterine transfusions, abnormal neurodevelopmental status was found in 5 (mild developmental delay in 3, severe delay in 2), and was not related to the severity of fetal anemia. Parvovirus infection may induce central nervous system damage.

Fetal CMV or toxoplasma infection can also present as hydrops. Maternal blood sample should be collected to check for specific antibodies. An amniotic fluid or fetal blood sample can be tested for the antigen. If fetal infection is confirmed, the finding of fetal hydrops means that the outlook for the pregnancy is very guarded with a high chance of a handicap.

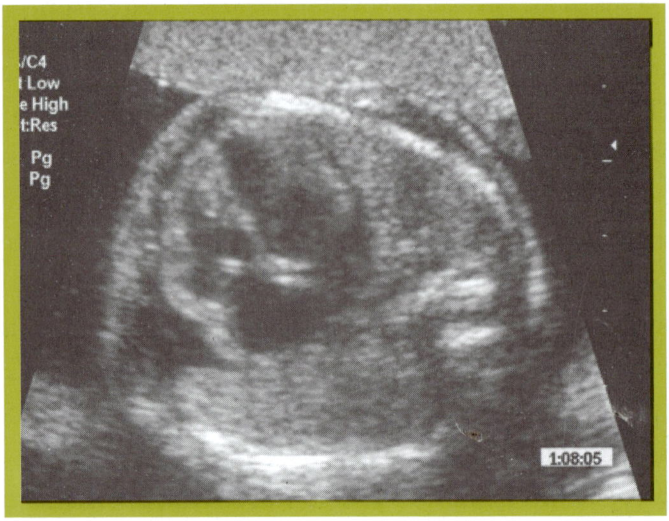

Figure 18.1: Fetal parvovirus infection; note the enlargement of the heart and presence of pleural and pericardial effusions.

Cardiac arrhythmias: Congenital tachy and bradyarrhythmias can lead to fetal hydrops. Congenital complete heart blocks can be caused by structural heart abnormalities such as left atrial isomerism or because anti-Ro/anti-La antibodies have destroyed the conduction system. The critical heart rate appears to be 55 BPM. If the heart rate falls below this rate, fetal hydrops will develop (Fig. 18.2).

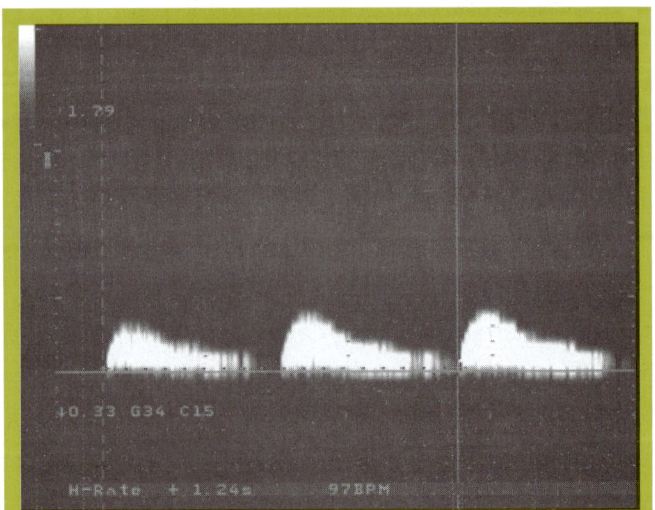

Figure 18.2: Complete heart block; note fetal bradycardia with a heart rate of 97 BPM.

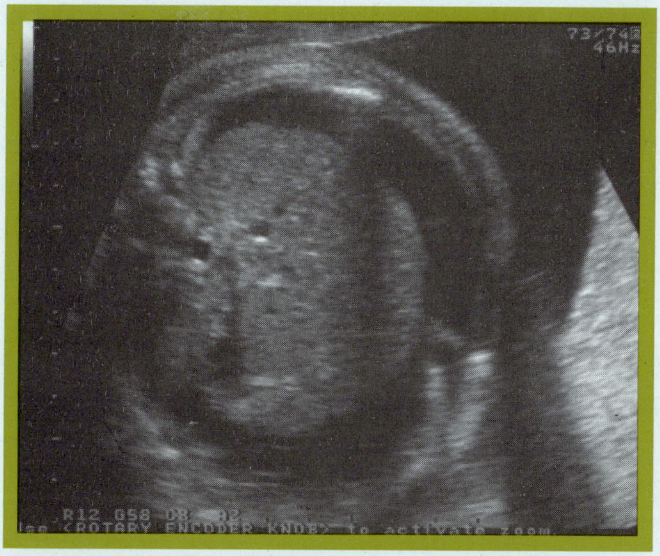

Figure 18.3: Hydrops in a case of fetal supraventricular tachycardia (SVT); the hydrops resolved on treatment and control of the heart rate.

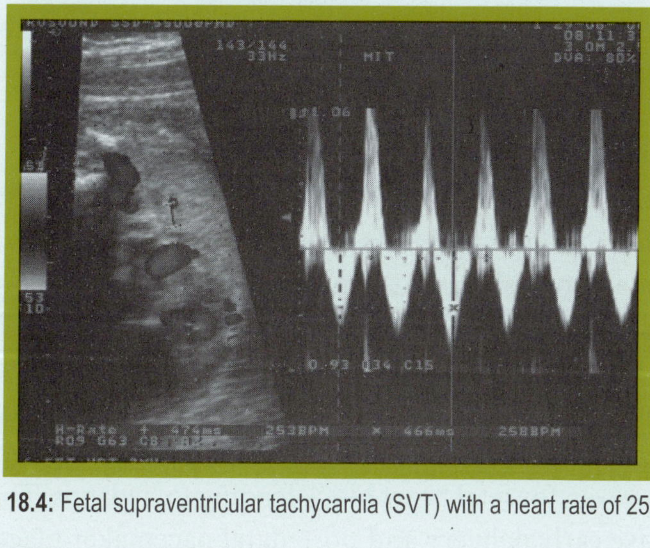

Figure 18.4: Fetal supraventricular tachycardia (SVT) with a heart rate of 258 BPM.

The outlook for hydrops due to bradycardia is poor. The heart rate responds poorly to pharmacological intervention. Hydrops resulting from fetal tachycardia has a much better outlook. Atrial flutter and supraventricular tachycardia (SVT) are common causes of fetal tachycardia leading to hydrops. Sustained fetal tachycardia with a 'critical' ventricular rate of over 210 BPM can result in fetal hydrops. Digoxin and flecainide have been used as first-line treatment for atrial flutter and SVT, respectively. Overall mortality of 8–9% has been reported (Figs 18.3 and 18.4).

Genetic or metabolic disorders: Several genetic or metabolic disorders such as storage disorders can lead to hydrops fetalis. Each of these conditions is very rare. A history of consanguinity is often present. There may be a history of fetal affliction. The diagnosis is usually based on postnatal or postmortem investigations. The outlook is guarded, as treatment options are very limited.

Hematological disorders: Genetic abnormalities such as congenital hemoglobinopathies (alpha thalassemia) can lead to fetal hydrops. Again, these are rare genetic abnormalities, and past history, family history or history of consanguinity may be present. Treatment options are limited and the outlook is guarded.

Complication of monochorionic twin pregnancy: Twin-to-twin transfusion syndrome (TTTS) and TRAP may lead to fetal hydrops. Typically, the recipient twin is hydropic in a TTTS setting, making it Stage IV TTTS. Refer to *Chapter 2, Twin Gestation and Invasive Testing* and *Chapter 15, Twin-to-Twin Transfusion Syndrome* for details.

Treatment of Hydrops Fetalis

The treatment is dependant on the cause. Effective treatment is available for fetal anemia, fetal tachyarrhythmias and twin-to-twin transfusion syndrome. Hydrops secondary to fetal anemia responds to correction of the anemia, usually with fetal transfusion.

Control of rapid fetal heart rate with transplacental pharmacotherapy is an effective way of correcting tachyarrhyhmias. Maternal digoxin or flecainide are drugs of choice. Rarely, direct fetal therapy is indicated. No effective treatment is available, however, for fetal heart block leading to hydrops. The only possible option is elective early delivery and post-natal pacemaker placement.

Refer to *Chapter 15, Twin-to-Twin Transfusion Syndrome* for details about the treatment of fetal hydrops resulting from TTTS.

If no cause can be identified, the condition is referred to as 'non-immune hydrops'. The prognosis is generally poor and is associated with approximately 80% mortality. In such cases, pregnancy termination (if legally permissible) is a valid option. The mother can develop a syndrome very similar to pre-eclampsia (Ballantyne syndrome/ Mirror syndrome). The pre-eclampsia can be very serious, and delivery may be indicated for maternal reasons.

Further Reading

- Krapp M, T Kohl, JM Simpson, GK Sharland, A Katalinic and U Gembruch. 2003. Review of diagnosis, treatment, and outcome of fetal atrial flutter compared with supraventricular tachycardia. *Heart* 89:913–17.
- Nagel HT, TR de Haan, FP Vandenbussche, D Oepkes and FJ Walther. 2007. Long-term outcome after fetal transfusion for hydrops associated with parvovirus B19 infection. *Obstet Gynecol* 109:42–47.
- Sohan K, SG Carroll, S de la Fuente, P Soothill and P Kyle. 2001. Analysis of outcome in hydrops fetalis in relation to gestational age at diagnosis, cause and treatment. *Acta Obstet Gynecol Scand* 80:726–30.

CHAPTER 19

OBSTRUCTIVE UROPATHY

Case: A pregnant woman was referred for a second opinion. A routine anomaly scan had been performed. The fetus appeared structurally normal. However, the urinary bladder was big and appeared to remain so even after careful scanning. The amniotic fluid volume was normal. The possibility of bladder outlet obstruction was raised, and the option of vesico-amniotic shunt placement was mooted.

After 16–18 weeks of pregnancy, fetal urine production makes a significant contribution to the amniotic fluid volume. Normal amniotic fluid volume suggests that fetal kidneys are functioning, and the fetus is able to void urine. Cases of bilateral renal agenesis show complete anhydramnios after 16–18 weeks' gestation. A finding of normal liquor volume in this case excludes complete bladder outlet obstruction. There may be incomplete or intermittent obstruction or no obstruction at all.

Embryology: Posterior urethral valves are structures that normally develop in the prostatic urethra between 6 and 8 weeks of gestation. Hypertrophy of these valves can lead to obstruction of the posterior urethra. The bladder is unable to empty itself. So the urine may reflux in both the ureters, and the pressure would eventually lead to permanent damage to the kidneys.

Urinary Bladder

In early pregnancy (11–14 weeks) a bladder measuring over 7 mm in largest diameter is considered a megacystis (Fig. 19.1). There is a high chance of a chromosomal abnormality or structural problem with the urinary tract, such as urethral atresia, in such cases. The implications of an enlarged bladder are not the same in the second trimester, however. Chromosomal abnormalities are rarely associated. Unfortunately, there is no definition for a 'normal' bladder size in the second

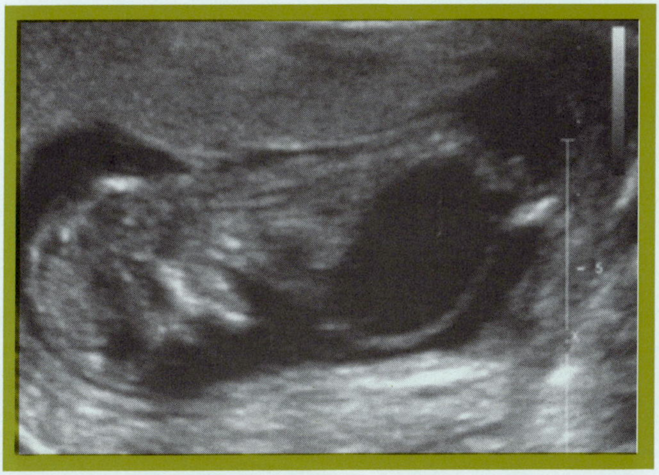

Figure 19.1: First trimester megacystis; note the size of the urinary bladder in relation to the CRL.

trimester or late pregnancy. An enlarged bladder is usually a subjective opinion. The urinary bladder is identified by the two umbilical arteries running on either side of it, on colour flow mapping.

The potential causes of enlarged urinary bladder are:

- Posterior urethral valves
- Bladder outlet obstruction/Urethral atresias
- Megacystis microcolon hypoperistalsis syndrome

Posterior urethral valves are typically over-diagnosed. They occur in male fetuses. The clinical course is variable, and onset may be any time from early intrauterine life to infancy. The valves as such cannot be seen. The dilated posterior urethra, however, can be seen, and along with a distended bladder, produces a 'keyhole' effect (Fig. 19.2). The diagnosis of posterior urethral valves is an inference. If the fetus is unable to void in the amniotic cavity, progressive reduction in amniotic fluid volume leading to complete anhydramnios by 18 weeks is the usual sequence of events.

Bladder outlet obstruction/atresia may be part of a cloacal abnormality. There is a high risk of genital abnormality. These fetuses may need reconstructive surgery on the external genitalia, and a gender reassignment may be involved.

Megacystis microcolon intestinal hypoperistalsis syndrome is a rare autosomal recessive genetic syndrome. Megacystis, variable degree of hydronephrosis and

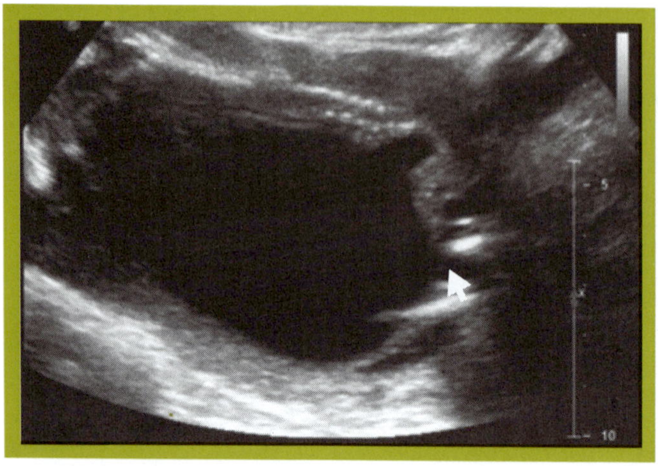

Figure 19.2: Megacystis due to posterior urethral valves. Note the dilated prostatic urethra (arrow). There is very little amniotic fluid around the fetus.

renal dysplasia, lax abdominal musculature and microcolon with dilated small bowel are the features. The bladder is big, but there is no obstruction to bladder outflow. The amniotic fluid quantity is normal or somewhat increased in these cases. There is marked female preponderance. The long-term outlook of affected babies is poor.

Treatment

Observation: Expectant management with serial scans is indicated when the amniotic fluid volume is relatively normal. Normal fluid volume beyond 18 weeks of pregnancy is indicative of continued renal function and the ability to void at least intermittently.

Vesicocentesis: Vesicocentesis, with decompression of the urinary bladder, sampling fetal urine and estimation of osmolality and electrolyte concentration in the fetal urine, was used as a predictor of renal function. This test has been used to select cases for antenatal intervention, where renal function is expected to be preserved. Repeated vesicocentesis has also been used in cases of obstructive uropathy till such time that a vesico-amniotic shunt becomes technically feasible. However, with the availability of medium- to long-term outcomes in cases of obstructive uropathy, the initial enthusiasm about antenatal intervention has not persisted (Fig. 19.3).

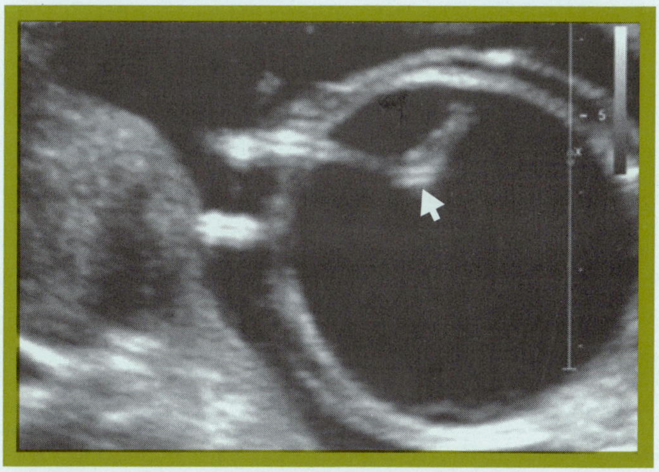

Figure 19.3: A double–pig-tailed vesico-amniotic shunt is in situ. The arrow shows the intravesical part of the shunt. Note the presence of amniotic fluid around the fetus.

Vesico-amniotic shunt: A vesico-amniotic shunt is placed for definitive treatment of obstructive uropathy. A double–pig-tailed shunt is used. However, the mother should be clearly told that shunt placement will not reverse pre-existing renal damage, but has the potential to limit further renal function deterioration. It can improve lung development, thereby reducing the risk of pulmonary hypoplasia. Placement is carried out under local anesthetic, and a special needle with a stent and a pusher are needed. Continuous ultrasound guidance is required. In cases where extreme oligohydramnios is present, antenatal amnio-infusion may have to be carried out prior to shunt placement. Care should be taken to avoid accidental injury to the umbilical arteries which lie on either side of the urinary bladder.

Termination of Pregnancy

This is indicated if additional abnormalities are present, or if there is ultrasound evidence of renal damage. Presence of echogenicities in the kidneys and evidence of oligohydramnios are suggestive of poor renal function.

For the pediatric surgeons, treatment of posterior urethral valves is fairly straightforward, and cystoscopic fulguration of the valves in the prostatic region of the urethra is all that is required. When this condition is suspected prenatally, management is rarely as straightforward.

A systematic review identified the lack of high-quality evidence to reliably inform clinical practice regarding prenatal bladder drainage in fetuses with ultrasonic evidence of lower urinary tract obstruction. The limited evidence available suggests that prenatal bladder drainage may improve perinatal survival in these fetuses, particularly those with poor predicted prognosis. However, the concern with vesico-amniotic shunting is pre-existing renal damage, which cannot be reversed and is difficult to quantify. Long-term follow-up of 34 children with prenatal treatment of obstructive uropathies was less encouraging. About 36% had renal failure requiring transplantation, and a further 21% had renal insufficiency. Urinary incontinence and surgery for bladder augmentation were other complications seen in this cohort.

Decompression of the fetal urinary bladder using a shunt at 13 + 5 weeks of pregnancy has been reported. The procedure may be technically possible, but it is too early to say if earlier decompression would result in better preservation of renal function.

Further Reading

- Clark TJ, W Martin, T Divakaran, M Whittle, M Kilby and K Khan. 2003. Prenatal bladder drainage in the management of fetal lower urinary tract obstruction: A systematic review and meta-analysis. *Obstet Gynecol* 102:367–82.
- Freedman A, M Johnson, C Smith, R Gonzalez and M Evans. 1999. Long-term outcome in children after antenatal intervention for obstructive uropathies. *Lancet* 354: 374–77.
- Kim S, H Won, J Shim, K Kim, P Lee and A Kim. 2005. Successful vesico-amniotic shunting of posterior urethral valves in the first trimester of pregnancy. *Ultrasound Obstet Gynecol* 26:666–668.
- Liao A, N Sebire, L Geerts, S Cicero and K Nicolaides. 2003. Megacystis at 10–14 weeks of gestation: Chromosomal defects and outcome according to bladder length. *Ultrasound Obstet Gynecol* 21: 338–41.

CHAPTER 20

ULTRASOUND DIAGNOSIS OF PLACENTA PREVIA

Case: A routine anomaly scan was carried out mid-pregnancy. The placenta was found to be situated covering the internal os. There was no history of vaginal bleeding. The sonographer informed the parents about the risk of placenta previa. The mother was considering taking a break from work and being on bed rest.

Definition

Traditionally, placenta previa has been defined as placental implantation in the lower uterine segment. The placental location was originally ascertained by clinical examination and digital palpation of the placental edge from the internal cervical os in the operating theatre. Consequently, several grades of placenta previa were described.

Grade 1: Lower edge of the placenta in the lower uterine segment but the lower edge not reaching the internal os.

Grade 2: Placental edge reaching the internal os but not covering it.

Grade 3: Placenta covering the internal os asymmetrically.

Grade 4: Placenta completely covering the internal os symmetrically.

Grades 1 and 2 were described as 'minor' previa, and Grades 3 and 4 as 'major' previa. The traditional classification of major and minor previa is arbitrary, and management of pregnancy and labour is not based on evidence. Currently, diagnosis of placenta previa is not based on digital examination of the placenta but on ultrasound scan. Despite the widespread and routine use of ultrasound to make the diagnosis of placenta previa, evidence-based classification and management strategies have failed to evolve over the years.

Screening for Placenta Previa

Currently, diagnosis is based on the findings of the ultrasound examination. It is common practice to perform an ultrasound examination mid-pregnancy—the so-called 'anomaly scan'. The placental location is routinely reported at this time. It is well-established that the use of transvaginal ultrasound is superior to that of transabdominal ultrasound in defining the relationship of the placental edge and the internal cervical os. The use of transvaginal ultrasound for the diagnosis of placenta previa is accurate as well as safe.

The relationship between the placental edge and the internal cervical os changes as the pregnancy advances. Use of ultrasound in the diagnosis of placenta previa overestimates the prevalence the earlier it is carried out in a pregnancy. Taipale et al screened 3696 women with transvaginal ultrasonography between 18 and 23 weeks. The placenta of 57 women (1.5%) was found to be either reaching or overlapping the internal cervical os (Fig. 20.1). Only 5 women (1.3 per 1000) were found to have placenta previa at delivery. In all 5 women, the placenta overlapped the internal cervical os by 15 mm or more in the mid-trimester scan.

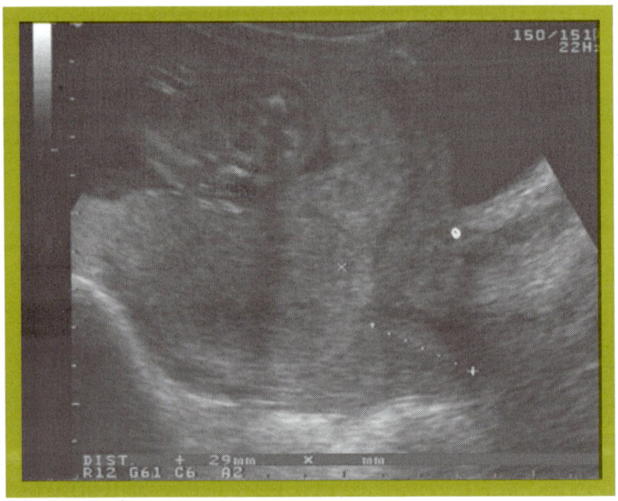

Figure 20.1: Mid-pregnancy ultrasound image showing placenta located over the internal os; the cervical canal measures 29 mm.

Several studies, including the abovementioned, show that unless the placental edge reaches at least the internal cervical os mid-pregnancy, placenta previa at term delivery is not likely to be encountered.

Most women who have a low placenta mid-pregnancy do not have placenta previa. This is because of 'placental migration'—differential placental development in the vascular upper segment at the expense of atrophy in the lower segment. In women with placental edge migration, the mean rate of migration was 5.4 mm per week in a study conducted by Oppenheimer et al.

Management of Low Placenta Mid-pregnancy

When should a placenta be termed 'low lying'? In asymptomatic women, unless the placental edge reaches or overlaps the internal os, the placenta should not be classified as low. If a woman has experienced vaginal bleeding, placental edge farther that 3.5 cm from the internal os is not associated with complications attributed to placenta previa.

If the mid-pregnancy scan shows an overlap of the placental edge (major placenta previa), the ultrasound scan should be repeated at 32 weeks. If the edge reached but did not overlap the internal os mid-pregnancy (minor placenta previa), the scan should be repeated at 36 weeks. A plan for delivery should be made at this stage. If major placenta previa persists in the 32 weeks' scan, the RCOG guidelines recommend hospitalisation and in-patient management even for asymptomatic women. However, this is not based on evidence, but rather on lack of evidence to support out-patient management of major placenta previa.

Plan for Delivery

Women with a placental edge that overlaps the internal os or is within 1 cm of the internal os require planned cesarean section, as the risk of major hemorrhage at delivery is high. Women with a placental edge over 2 cm from the internal os should be encouraged to attempt a normal birth as there is >60% chance of vaginal birth. Cases with an internal os–placental edge of 2.0–3.5 cm should still be called 'low lying placenta' as a risk of excessive bleeding after delivery still exists. The optimal management of women with a placental edge–internal os distance between 1 and 2 cm is unclear. A planned cesarean section is probably

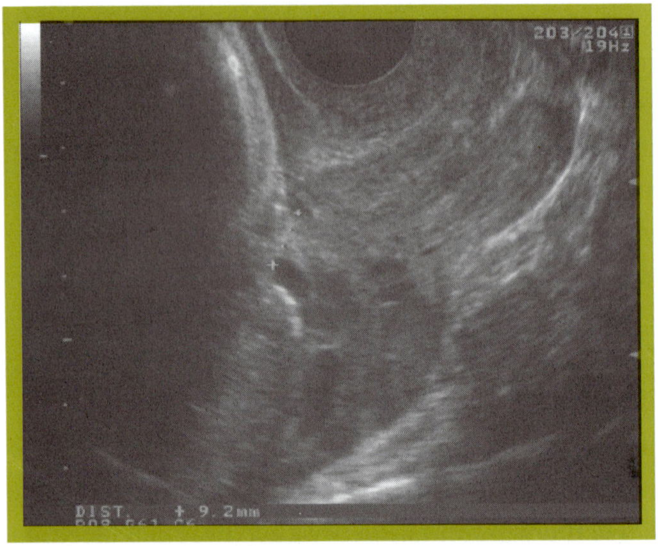

Figure 20.2: Transvaginal scan at 38 weeks showing the internal os–placental edge distance of 9.2 mm; an elective cesarean section was planned.

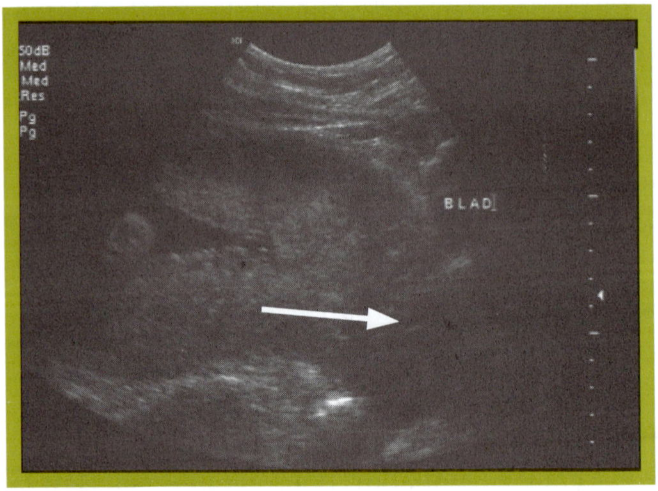

Figure 20.3: Major placenta previa located symmetrically over the internal os (arrow).

the safest option in these cases. The risk of postpartum hemorrhage remains high even in cases of placenta previa selected for a vaginal birth attempt. Provision of adequate cross-matched blood should not be forgotten (Figs 20.2 and 20.3).

and a single umbilical artery had other ultrasonically detected abnormalities. Thus the risk of chromosomal abnormalities in the absence of other detectable abnormalities or markers appears to be low. Karyotyping should be offered if other markers or abnormalities are seen on the scan.

Risk of associated structural abnormalities

Benirschke, the well-known perinatal pathologist, made a plea for examination of the placenta and the umbilical cord after delivery in the era prior to wide availability of ultrasound evaluation of the fetus. The basis was a high incidence of structural abnormalities when the umbilical cord revealed only two vessels. This has changed radically with the availability of high-definition ultrasound for fetal evaluation. Many fetuses with a single umbilical artery also show structural abnormalities on the scan. Not all structural abnormalities are detected antenatally, however. In a study reporting 61 cases with a single umbilical artery, 23 were thought to have no associated abnormalities at prenatal evaluation. Seven of these 23 (30.4%) were found to have structural defects after birth (three cases with cardiac defects, three with renal abnormalities and one with a limb defect). A careful and thorough assessment of the fetus for structural abnormalities should be done when a two-vessel cord is diagnosed on prenatal ultrasound assessment.

Growth restriction

There is a theoretical concern that one umbilical artery instead of the normally seen two may lead to interference with placental gas exchange and transfer of nutrients. Indeed, there are some reports of a higher incidence of fetal growth restriction in fetuses with a two-vessel cord. However, it is now increasingly becoming clear that in the absence of associated abnormalities on the ultrasound, the prevalence of fetal growth restriction in cases of single umbilical artery is not different from those with three vessels. Volumetric flow study has demonstrated that the volume of blood carried by a single umbilical artery is twice that of each of the two umbilical arteries.

If the fetus is small for gestational age, umbilical artery Doppler should be used with caution. While a high resistance is indicative of placental insufficiency, normal Doppler indices cannot be reassuring. Fetuses with a single umbilical artery typically demonstrate low pulsatile index (PI) and resistance index (RI) for the gestation using the standard reference range derived from the normal population. On the other hand, the MCA Doppler indices in fetuses with SUI have a distribution similar to that of normal fetuses throughout gestation. Fetal MCA Doppler indices can probably be interpreted in the same way in fetuses with SUI as for fetuses with a three-vessel cord.

Management of a Fetus with a Single Umbilical Artery

In many cases, a single umbilical artery is identified subsequent to detection of another major structural defect. A thorough ultrasound assessment should be made when a single umbilical artery is detected. Karyotyping should be considered, particularly if other abnormalities have been seen. It is worthwhile arranging follow-up scans at 28 and 34 weeks to check fetal growth. If no structural abnormalities are seen, the parents should be reassured. The risk of complications for the pregnancy or the baby is low in such cases.

Further Reading

- Lubusky M, I Dhaifalah, M Prochazka, J Hyjanek, I Mickova, K Vomackova and J Santavy. 2007. Single umbilical artery and its siding in the second trimester of pregnancy: Relation to chromosomal defects. *Prenat Diagn* 27:327–31.
- Predanic M, SC Perni, A Friedman, FA Chervenak and ST Chasen. 2005. Fetal growth assessment and neonatal birth weight in fetuses with an isolated single umbilical artery. *Obstet Gynecol* 105:1093–97.

CHAPTER 22

FACIAL CLEFT

Case: A routine anomaly scan was carried out mid-pregnancy. The ultrasonographer noticed a unilateral cleft lip and alveolus in the fetus. No additional anomalies were identified. It was not clear whether or not amniocentesis should be carried out for karyotype.

Cleft lip with or without palate occurs in approximately 1:700 fetuses. Cleft lip may or may not be associated with a cleft in the alveolus (gum) and the hard palate. Isolated cleft of the soft palate is a distinct entity and is often associated with genetic syndromes. A cleft in the upper lip can be seen on the scan (Fig. 22.1), whereas the palate is almost impossible to view on the scan. Facial clefts can be simple or complex. The most common time for the identification (or exclusion) of facial cleft is at the time of an anomaly scan, which is carried out at around 20 weeks of pregnancy. It is possible to diagnose facial cleft earlier, but definitive diagnosis may be difficult. Facial cleft has been diagnosed at 11–14 weeks, but this is usually in cases where there is a high degree of suspicion (previous or family history of facial cleft).

Simple Cleft

A paramedian cleft of the lip and the alveolus is a relatively common congenital abnormality. The usual location is at the junction of the philtrum and lateral aspect of the upper lip. Sometimes the cleft can be bilateral, on both sides (Figs 22.2 and 22.3). A simple cleft is usually not associated with other abnormalities or abnormal karyotype. There may be a family history of facial cleft. There are

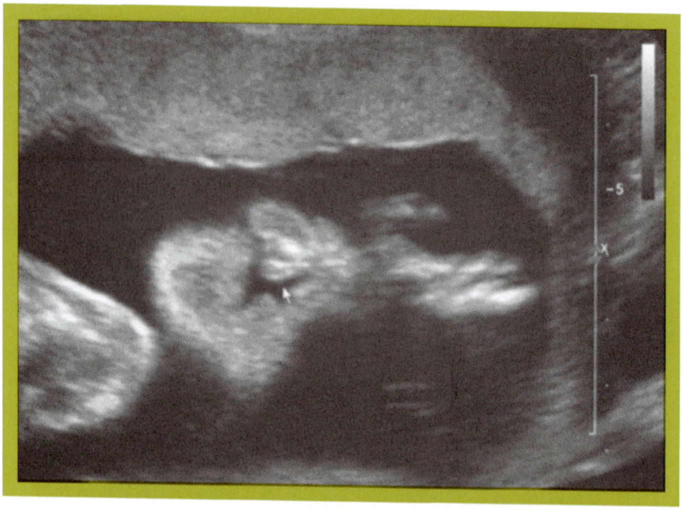

Figure 22.1: Ultrasound scan showing a unilateral cleft lip

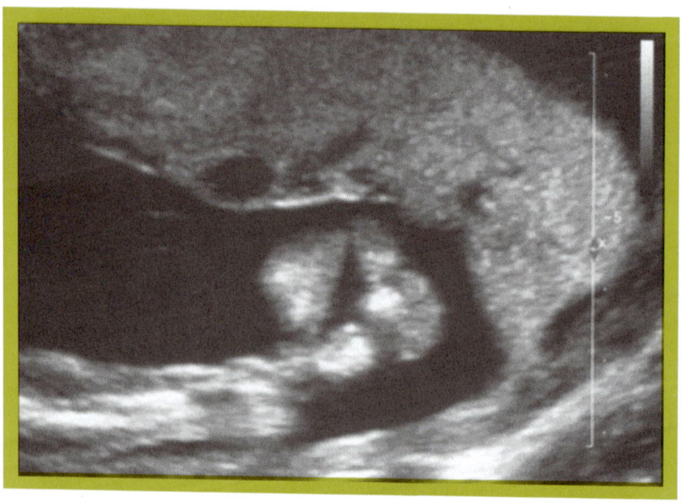

Figure 22.2: Ultrasound scan showing bilateral cleft in the upper lip

many genetic syndromes associated with cleft lip and alveolus, such as oro-facio-digital syndrome and Varadi–Papp syndrome.

In a large European study, 751 cases with facial cleft were reported. Prenatal diagnosis was made in 65 of 366 cases (18%) with an isolated malformation. The sensitivity was better (52%) in cases with chromosomal abnormalities. The prenatal diagnosis of cleft palate was made in 13 of 198 cases (6.5%).

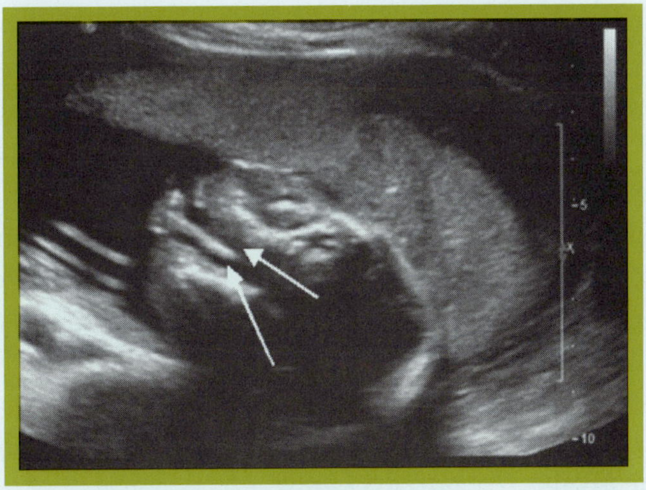

Figure 22.3: Ultrasound scan of the same fetus as in Fig. 22.2. Bilateral defect in the palate is shown (arrows).

The sensitivity of centres with skilled operators is better than in this report. A sensitivity of 75% has been reported for isolated facial clefts.

A 3D ultrasound may be used for prenatal visualisation of the cleft lip (Fig. 22.4). The palate may be assessed using sequential scrolling of the view bar through the acquired 3D volume. However, shadowing from surrounding bones often restricts visualisation. The technique of 'reverse face view' has been proposed

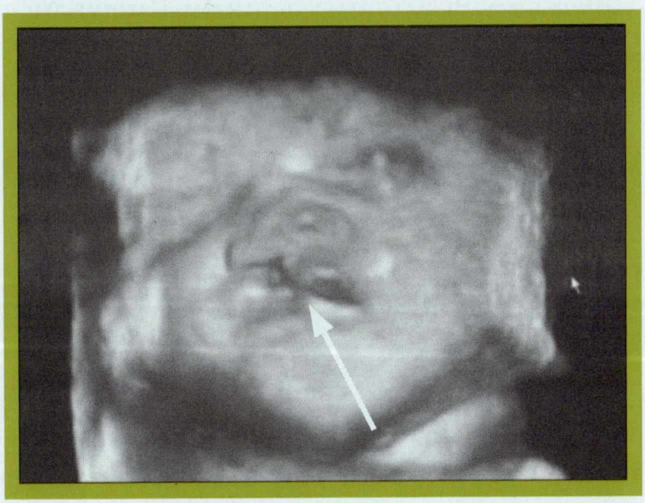

Figure 22.4: A 3D ultrasound scan showing a right-sided paramedian cleft in the upper lip

to make an accurate prenatal diagnosis of cleft palate. In the conventional 3D technique, the view bar is scrolled from the lips to the alveolar ridge and the palate. In the 'reverse face view' technique, a frontal view of the face is made, and the face rotated 180° before scrolling the view bar. This was intended to avoid shadowing of the image and to provide clearer pictures of the palate.

There is no evidence to suggest that availability of 3D ultrasound will improve the sensitivity of prenatal diagnosis of isolated cleft lip/palate. However, the 3D ultrasound image of the affected fetus provides an opportunity for the parents to understand the defect, come to terms with it, and mentally be better prepared for the arrival of the newborn.

What should the prospective parents know?

Although facial cleft can be repaired with little residual disability, it is very disturbing for the parents. The major concerns are cosmetic, feeding, dentition and speech. The immediate concern for doctors is feeding. A defect in the palate means that the baby will be unable to suck and swallow. Breastfeeding will not be possible, but breast milk can be administered until the defect in the palate is repaired.

The different medical specialties involved in managing the cleft lip may have conflicting interests. Dentists would want to operate as late as possible, because the operation would interfere with secondary dentition. Parents are more concerned about the facial appearance and would prefer an early repair. The compromise is a repair carried out in stages. Palatine soft-tissue defects are closed early to allow normal feeding. The bony gap is then closed much later.

Parents are usually provided with written information produced by the Cleft Lip and Palate Association (CLAPA). The CLAPA website (www.clapa.com) is also very informative.

Complex Cleft

A midline cleft, facial cleft that is not characteristic or facial cleft with presence of other ultrasound markers should be classified as a complex cleft (Fig. 22.5). A midline cleft is often associated with holoprocencephaly, a major abnormality of the central nervous system. Trisomy 13 is a common cause. Attention should be paid to the other facial structures and the ultrasound appearance of the fetal brain.

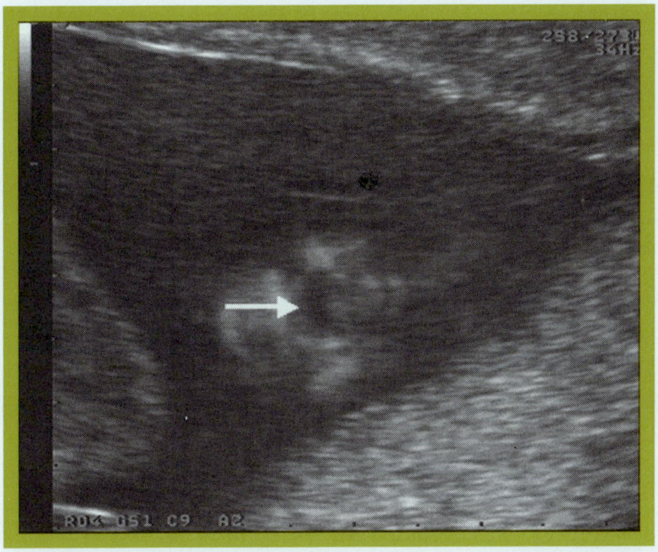

Figure 22.5: Ultrasound scan showing a midline facial cleft (arrow)

The outlook in complex facial cleft is much more guarded. Other abnormalities are often associated. History of consanguinity, past history of affected fetuses or family history is suggestive of an underlying genetic syndrome.

Should amniocentesis be offered in cases of prenatally diagnosed facial clefts?

The decision to carry out amniocentesis will depend on the perceived risk of chromosomal abnormality. This is influenced by several factors such as the mother's age, prior nuchal translucency screening, presence of other ultrasound soft markers of chromosomal abnormality and the parents' views and expectations. For isolated paramedian cleft lip/alveolus with no additional markers, there is little to recommend amniocentesis. On the other hand, invasive prenatal diagnosis should strongly be considered in complex clefts.

Further Reading

- Campbell S, C Lees, G Moscoso and P Hall. 2005. Ultrasound antenatal diagnosis of cleft palate by a new technique: The 3D 'reverse face' view. *Ultrasound Obstet Gynecol* 25:12–18.

Further Reading

- Clementi M, R Tenconi, F Bianchi and C Stoll. 2000. Evaluation of prenatal diagnosis of cleft lip with or without cleft palate and cleft palate by ultrasound: Experience from 20 European registries. EUROSCAN study group. *Prenat Diagn* 20:870–75.
- Wayne C, K Cook, S Sairam, B Hollis and B Thilaganathan. 2002. Sensitivity and accuracy of routine antenatal ultrasound screening for isolated facial clefts. *Br J Radiol* 75:584–89.

CHAPTER 23

IRREGULAR HEART RHYTHM ON FETAL HEART AUSCULTATION

Case: A woman in her second pregnancy underwent a routine antenatal checkup in the antenatal clinic. The midwife palpated the abdomen and declared that all was well. However, when the fetal heart was auscultated, a clear irregularity in rhythm was observed. The mother was referred to the Fetal Medicine department for an urgent assessment of the fetal heart.

Types of Arrhythmias

- Irregular heart beat
    - Atrial/Supraventricular premature beat
    - Ventricular premature beat
    - Atrio-ventricular block
- Tachyarrhythmias
    - Sinus tachycardia
    - Supraventricular tachycardia (SVT)
    - Atrial flutter/fibrillation with or without block
- Bradyarrhythmias
    - Sinus bradycardia
    - Atrio-ventricular block

Diagnostic Tools

Although fetal ECG can be obtained non-invasively through the maternal abdomen, the fetal electrical signals are very weak compared to maternal

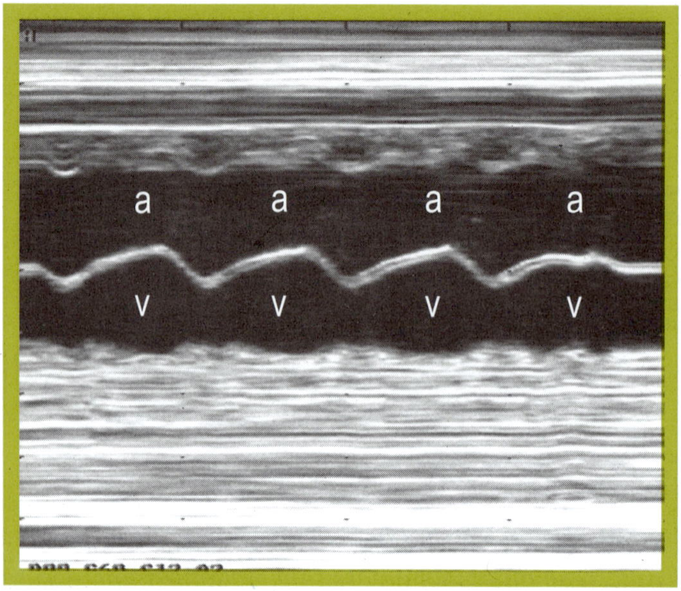

Figure 23.1: Normal atrio-ventricular movement on M-mode ultrasound scan

signals. The problem of electrical 'noise' and obtaining pure electrical signals clear enough to identify the components of the ECG continue to exist. The technique is still not useful in clinical practice. M-mode imaging and pulsed wave Doppler ultrasound are used to identify mechanical events known to be associated with electrical components of the ECG. The P wave of the ECG corresponds to atrial contraction, and the QRS complex to ventricular contraction. The time duration between the atrial and ventricular contractions corresponds to the P-R interval. Unfortunately, the T wave has no mechanical activity associated with it and cannot be identified using ultrasound.

M-mode imaging shows movement of all the structures in the path of the cursor with time. A normal M-mode image shows atrial and ventricular wall motion. The cursor should pass through the atrial and ventricular wall simultaneously. The time interval between the atrial and ventricular contractions is referred to as the A-V interval, whereas the interval between a ventricular contraction and the next atrial contraction is the V-A interval. Figure 23.1 shows normal atrio-ventricular movement.

Pulsed wave Doppler requires simultaneous arterial and venous signals because atrial contractions can be identified on venous flow, whereas ventricular

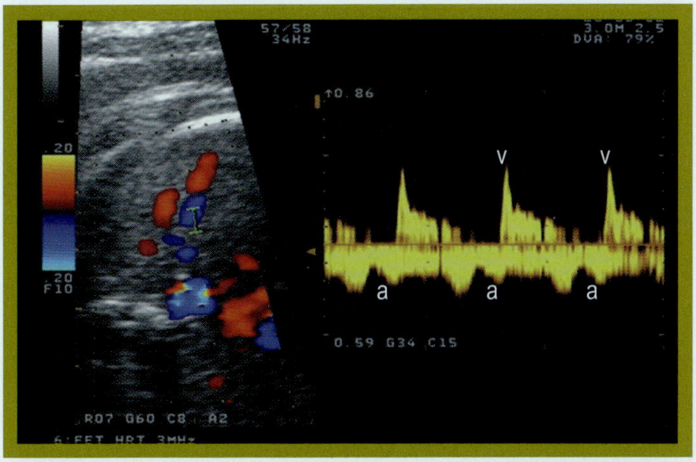

Figure 23.2: Pulmonary artery and vein pulsed wave Doppler evaluation. Atrial contractions (a) are reflected in the venous flow and ventricular contractions (v) in the arterial flow.

contractions are identified only on arterial signal. Unfortunately, the aorta and vena cava are not physically close to each other, and simultaneous recording of the arterio-venous waveforms is not possible. Pulmonary vasculature provides a unique opportunity where waveforms in the pulmonary artery and vein can be recorded simultaneously. Figure 23.2 shows a normal sinus rhythm as evaluated on pulmonary artery and vein pulsed wave Doppler.

Premature Beats

These are the commonest cause of fetal arrhythmias, with atrial premature beats being more common than ventricular premature beats.

Figures 23.3 and 23.4 show the assessment of premature beats by the M-mode and pulsed wave Doppler techniques.

The outlook for premature beats is very good, and the irregularity in heart rhythm disappears either before or after delivery in a large majority of cases. On rare occasions, successive premature beats may trigger a re-entry phenomenon, and an SVT may result. Three or more successive premature beats qualify to be termed 'tachycardia' although they are of very short duration. Premature beats rarely require intervention, apart from reassurance. In a small proportion of cases, premature beats in tandem may trigger sustained tachyarrhythmia. Successive (two, three or more in a row) premature beats or frequent (more than five in one minute) beats require surveillance to find out if sustained tachycardia develops.

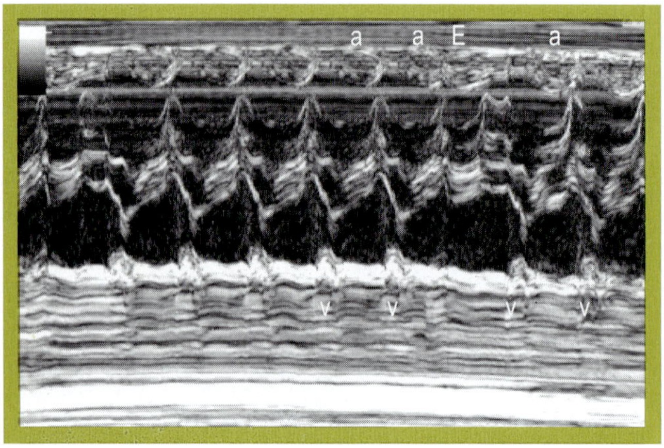

Figure 23.3: M-mode echocardiography. Atrial contractions (a) are followed by ventricular contractions (v). An atrial ectopic contraction (E) is not followed by a ventricular contraction.

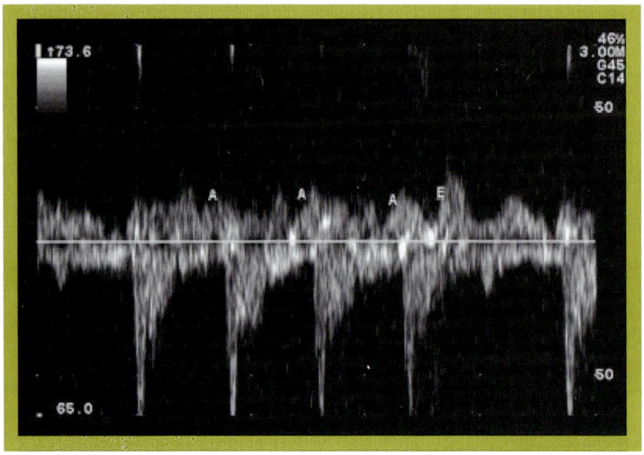

Figure 23.4: Simultaneous recording of the pulmonary artery and vein. Atrial contractions (A) are followed by ventricular contractions (below the baseline). A premature atrial contraction (E) is not followed by a ventricular contraction.

The irregularity of the rhythm is often persistent on routine auscultation of the fetal heart. Follow-up assessment is required only if the heart rate is less than 100 or more than 200, or if there are concerns with fetal movement. The baby also needs an ECG after birth, if the heart rhythm remains abnormal.

Fetal Tachycardias

Sustained fetal heart rate above 180 BPM represents fetal tachycardia. Maternal pyrexia, medications (beta sympathomimetic agents such as asthma medicines),

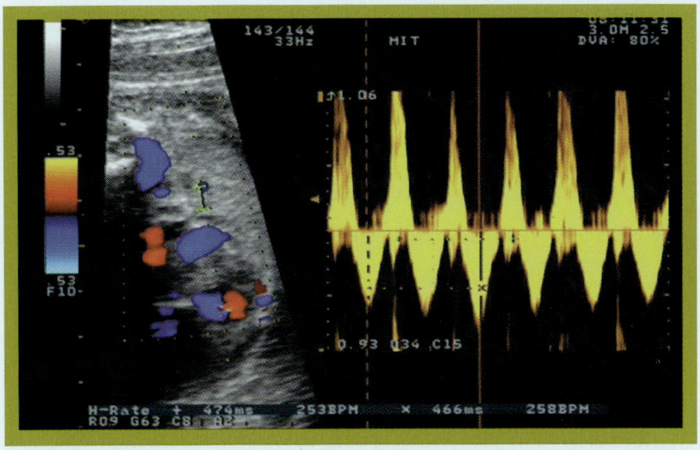

Figure 23.5: Simultaneous recording of pulmonary artery (above the baseline) and pulmonary vein (below the baseline) waveforms using pulsed wave Doppler. Note 1:1 conduction and a heart rate of 258 BPM.

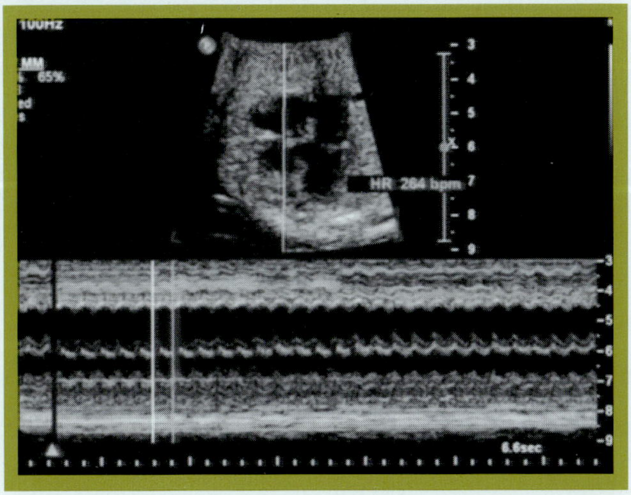

Figure 23.6: Use of M-mode ultrasound in the demonstration of SVT with a heart rate of 264 BPM.

sustained fetal activity and fetal hyperthyroidism are some of the causes of sinus tachycardia. The fetal heart rate usually returns to normal once the causative factor has been removed.

Supraventricular tachycardia (SVT) and atrial flutter (AF) are the two common reasons for sustained fetal tachycardia, in the proportion of 3:1 by frequency. AF is detected at a significantly later gestational age than SVT (30 and 28 weeks, respectively).

Figures 23.5 and 23.6 show the evaluation of SVT and AF using the M-mode imaging and pulsed wave Doppler techniques.

Very rapid heart rate leads to shortening of the ventricular filling time. It may also lead to increased atrial and venous pressures and congestive heart failure, resulting in hydrops fetalis. The critical rate appears to be 210 BPM, above which hydrops develops if the rate is sustained. Ultrasound markers of clinical progression are cardiomegaly, appearance of A-V regurgitation, dilated fetal veins, hydrops, polyhydramnios and placental enlargement.

Approximately 40% of fetuses show features of hydrops at initial presentation. In a large series, the mortality rate was reported to be 8–9%. Maternal administration of digoxin is the first line therapy in cases of SVT and AF. Transplacental passage of digoxin is often unsatisfactory in hydrops and placental edema. Flecainide, a second line drug, is rapidly becoming the drug of choice for the treatment of SVT/AF. The transplacental transfer of flecainide is satisfactory even in the presence of placental edema. Maternal admission and ECG, with drug level monitoring, is required for drug treatment as the therapeutic window is narrow and maternal toxicity can easily occur. If the heart rhythm is successfully converted to sinus, vaginal birth may be acheived. The newborn needs an ECG and echocardiography after birth. Many babies do not require flecainide therapy.

Fetal Bradyarrhythmias

Blocked atrial premature beats can potentially halve the ventricular rate if the alternate atrial signal is premature. In keeping with all other atrial premature beats, this abnormality is benign and disappears spontaneously in a large majority of cases. Atrio-ventricular block of varying degree has a more guarded prognosis. The most severe of these is a complete A-V block. The ventricles have a spontaneous rate which is relatively fixed. The critical ventricular rate appears to be 55 BPM. Rates below this limit are usually associated with cardiac failure and hydrops.

Some cases of complete heart block result from maternal anti-Ro/La antibodies. These antibodies can be transferred across the placenta and interfere with the conduction system between the AV node and bundle of His, leading to electrical disassociation. Immune-mediated CHB typically occurs at

20–24 weeks of pregnancy. Structural heart abnormalities such as congenitally corrected transposition of the great arteries and heterotaxy syndromes (left atrial isomerism) can also lead to a complete A-V block. Majority of the cases without a structural heart abnormality will show presence of auto-antibodies in maternal serum.

The outlook of fetuses with complete heart block and hydrops is guarded, as there is no known prenatal intervention. Maternal beta sympathomimetic therapy in an attempt to increase fetal heart rate has only produced inconclusive results. In the group with auto-antibodies, administration of steroids is of no use once complete heart block occurs. Use of steroids to prevent progression of a first-degree block to CHB in mothers with auto-antibodies is controversial and unproven.

Survival of fetuses with a structural abnormality is much worse than in those that are structurally normal. Overall survival is reported to be 18% and 75%, respectively. If there is no hydrops, no prenatal intervention is required, although intrapartum monitoring using CTG is impossible because of the abnormal heart rate. Moreover, fetal hypoxia may not lead to fetal heart rate abnormalities in fetuses with a complete heart block. Some of these fetuses will require postnatal placement of a permanent pacemaker.

Further Reading

- Carvalho JS, F Prefumo, V Ciardelli, S Sairam, A Bhide and EA Shinebourne. 2007. Evaluation of fetal arrhythmias from simultaneous pulsed wave Doppler in pulmonary artery and vein. *Heart* 93:1448–53.
- Friedman D and J Buyon. 2005. Complete atrioventricular block diagnosed prenatally: Anything new on the block? *Ultrasound Obstet Gynecol* 26:2–3.
- Krapp M, T Kohl, J Simpson, G Sharland, A Katalinic and U Gembruch. 2003. Review of diagnosis, treatment, and outcome of fetal atrial flutter compared with supraventricular tachycardia. *Heart* 89:913–17.

Index